MEDICAL MIRTHOLOGY

Finding humor in medical practice

MORRIS D. CHARENDOFF

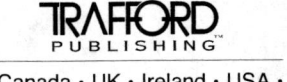

· Canada · UK · Ireland · USA ·

© Copyright 2006 Morris D. Charendoff. .
All rights reserved. No part of this publication may be reproduced, stored in a retrieval system, or transmitted, in any form or by any means, electronic, mechanical, photocopying, recording, or otherwise, without the written prior permission of the author.
Note for Librarians: A cataloguing record for this book is available from Library and Archives Canada at www.collectionscanada.ca/amicus/index-e.html
ISBN 1-4120-7801-6

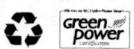

Printed in Victoria, BC, Canada. Printed on paper with minimum 30% recycled fibre. Trafford's print shop runs on "green energy" from solar, wind and other environmentally-friendly power sources.

TRAFFORD
PUBLISHING

Offices in Canada, USA, Ireland and UK
This book was published *on-demand* in cooperation with Trafford Publishing. On-demand publishing is a unique process and service of making a book available for retail sale to the public taking advantage of on-demand manufacturing and Internet marketing. On-demand publishing includes promotions, retail sales, manufacturing, order fulfilment, accounting and collecting royalties on behalf of the author.

Book sales for North America and international:
Trafford Publishing, 6E–2333 Government St.,
Victoria, BC V8T 4P4 CANADA
phone 250 383 6864 (toll-free 1 888 232 4444)
fax 250 383 6804; email to orders@trafford.com

Book sales in Europe:
Trafford Publishing (UK) Limited, 9 Park End Street, 2nd Floor
Oxford, UK OX1 1HH UNITED KINGDOM
phone 44 (0)1865 722 113 (local rate 0845 230 9601)
facsimile 44 (0)1865 722 868; info.uk@trafford.com

Order online at:
trafford.com/05-2698
10 9 8 7 6

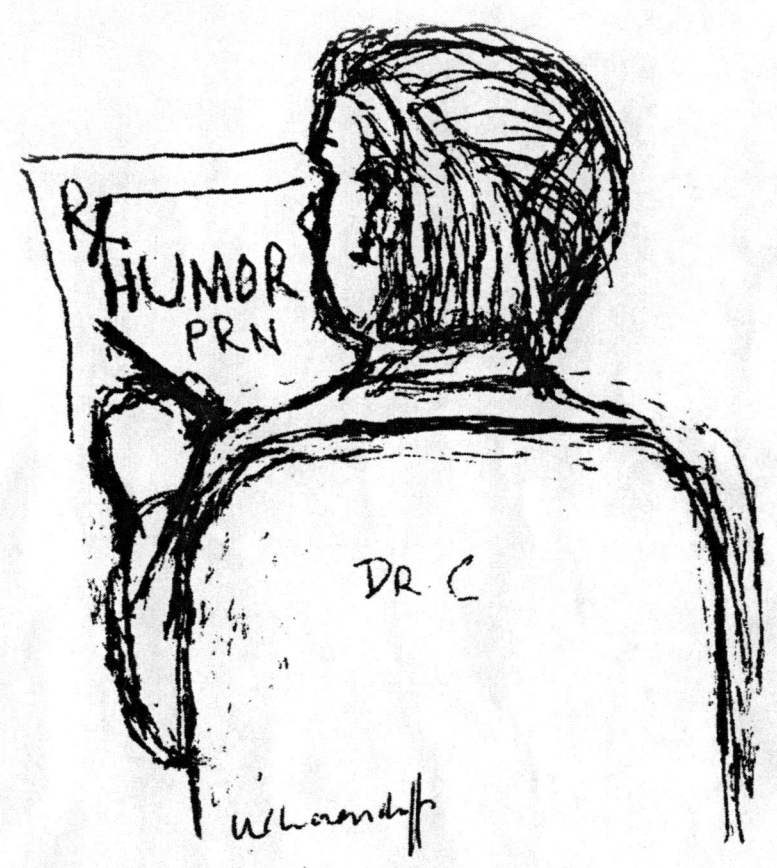

Dedication

To my wife, Hudy, who has the best sense of humor of all and who has laughed with and not at me for many years now.

To my children Jay, Debbi and Susan.

Finally, to all those patients and colleagues who wittingly or otherwise provided me with an abundance of material.

Acknowledgements

I owe a debt of gratitude to my colleagues for their camaraderie and support, and for sharing their stories with me over the years. I'd like to thank specifically David Rapoport, a Toronto family physician whose avocation is writing medical humor, and Ken Shonk whose Kitchener, Ontario, medical practice successfully incorporates the use of humor and laughter.

I would like to thank Janice Kretchman for sharing her editorial and organizational skills and Susan Charendoff-Stein for the biographical sketch of her father and her help in proof-reading this book. Thanks also go to Stewart Stein for his work designing the cover and to my wife, Hudy, for the use of her collage.

Finally, a sincere thanks to all who contributed in many other ways and encouraged me to write this book.

Table of Contents

Introduction	11
Getting to Know You	13
The Price and Power of Fame	19
Adventures with My Colleagues	29
Medical School (Mis)Adventures	35
Hospitals	41
Patients, Patient or Otherwise	51
Medical Miscellanae	67
Afterlaughs	79

Introduction

I suppose I became aware of the humor daily life has to offer many years ago.

When I was 7 years old, I sold copies of the Toronto Daily Star at the corner of Spadina and Bloor in downtown Toronto. My daily quota was 25 papers, at a cost of 2 cents each. I had paid 1 cent apiece, and so if I sold the entire quota I would earn 25 cents.

One day in the middle of winter, the weather was brutally cold – about -30 degrees Fahrenheit. I was freezing, and it was too cold even for most customers to stop. Most, yes, but after a time a car did pull up at my location. The driver honked to get my attention and beckoned me to come over.

It was Uncle Dave.

"Moishe, I want to buy all your papers so you can go home. It's too cold to be out."

"I'm sorry uncle. Only one paper to a customer."

I was young and stubborn, and remained at my corner until all the papers were sold. And then laughed about it later on.

If you ever thought your laughter was a mere involuntary reaction to something you found amusing, you have been greatly misled. Laughter is an altogether more serious undertaking and there is a long history in the belief a humorous outlook can help both prevent and cure disease.

Henri de Mondeville (1260-1320), medieval professor of surgery, wrote "The surgeon must forbid anger, hatred and sadness in the patient and remind him the body grows fat from joy and thin from sadness."

The practice of keeping court fools or jesters is regarded as a medieval institution. Among the least recognized function of the jesters was their role in maintaining the physical and emotional health of the monarch.

Thomas Fuller, writing in the beginning of the 17th century comments, "Mirth is the best cardio against the consumption of the spirit."

MEDICAL MIRTHOLOGY *(Finding Humor in Medical Practice)*

In his 1621 "Anatomy of Melancholy," Robert Burton wrote "mirth purges the blood, confirms health, causeth a fresh pleasing and fine color, prolongs life... makes the body young, lively and fit for any manner of employment."

In "Tom Sawyer" Mark Twain writes "the old man laughed loud and joyously, shook up the details of his anatomy from head to foot and ended by saying that such laughter was money in a man's pocket because it cut down the doctor's bill like everything."

In "Medical Mirthology" I have collected authentic humorous incidents from medical school, internship and my practice itself. These experiences have been richly rewarding, and have had a significant impact on my personality and outlook.

It did not occur to me at the time they would one day become a book.

As a physician I am always interacting with people, frequently at the most vulnerable times in their lives. In spite of that I have found there is a place for humor, and that it has a salutary effect.

Medical Mirthology is a book about humor in medicine, and the beneficial effects of laughter on health. It is not another joke book about doctors.

Much of the material is from my own personal practice and experience. All the stories are authentic.

I hope you find the contents amusing and enjoyable. Even more important than that, I hope you benefit physiologically and emotionally.

Doctors often don't like to use humor for fear of offending, and so risk appearing emotionless and uncaring. However humor, properly used, is a most effective forms of communication.

You can be the most knowledgeable physician in the world but if you are not able to relate to your patients, you are not doing them the most good.

"Take your job seriously, but yourself lightly."

Getting to Know You

"A merry heart doeth good like a medicine but a broken spirit dryeth the bone."
~ Proverbs 17:22 ~

History Taking

Obtaining information from a patient is an art. Sometimes even when you think you are asking the right questions you don't get the right answers. It took me quite a while to develop my technique, and sometimes it was a frustrating learning experience.

I can best illustrate this by outlining a particular incident from my earlier years, when I was attempting to take a history from a middleage Jewish lady...

Doctor: Good morning, I am Dr. Charendoff. How are you?
Patient: Don't ask.
Doctor: What is the reason you are here?
Patient: My doctor sent me.
Doctor: How did you get to me?
Patient: I made an appointment.
Doctor: I mean, what brought you here?
Patient: I took a bus first and then walked from the corner.
Doctor: What is your problem?
Patient: My doctor knows all about it.
Doctor: Why did he send you here?
Patient: He said you are a good doctor.
Doctor: All right then. Do you have any complaints?
Patient: I never complain. My doctor knows that.
Doctor: Do you have any pain?
Patient: Don't ask.

MEDICAL MIRTHOLOGY *(Finding Humor in Medical Practice)*

Doctor: Where is your pain?
Patient: All over.
(making a big circle with her hand, indicating her entire body)
Doctor: Can you be more specific? Show me where it hurts with one finger.
Patient: Yes I can.
(making the same circle, this time with one finger)
Doctor: Is the pain bad?
Patient: Don't ask.
Doctor: How bad?
Patient: All my enemies should have such pain.
Doctor: What kind of pain is it?
Patient: It's the same pain as my neighbour has. She came to you too.
Doctor: When did this pain start?
Patient: Three months after my daughter gave birth.
Doctor: And when was that?
Patient: Six months after we moved into our apartment.
Doctor: When do you have the pain?
Patient: All the time, it never stops. Night and day.
Doctor: The pain is constant?
Patient: All my enemies should have such pain.
Doctor: What makes the pain worse?
Patient: My husband.
Following the examination, it was determined an operation was indicated. We continued:
Doctor: I believe you could be helped by an operation.
Patient: All right Dr. Charendoff. Who would you suggest should do it?
Doctor: Don't ask.

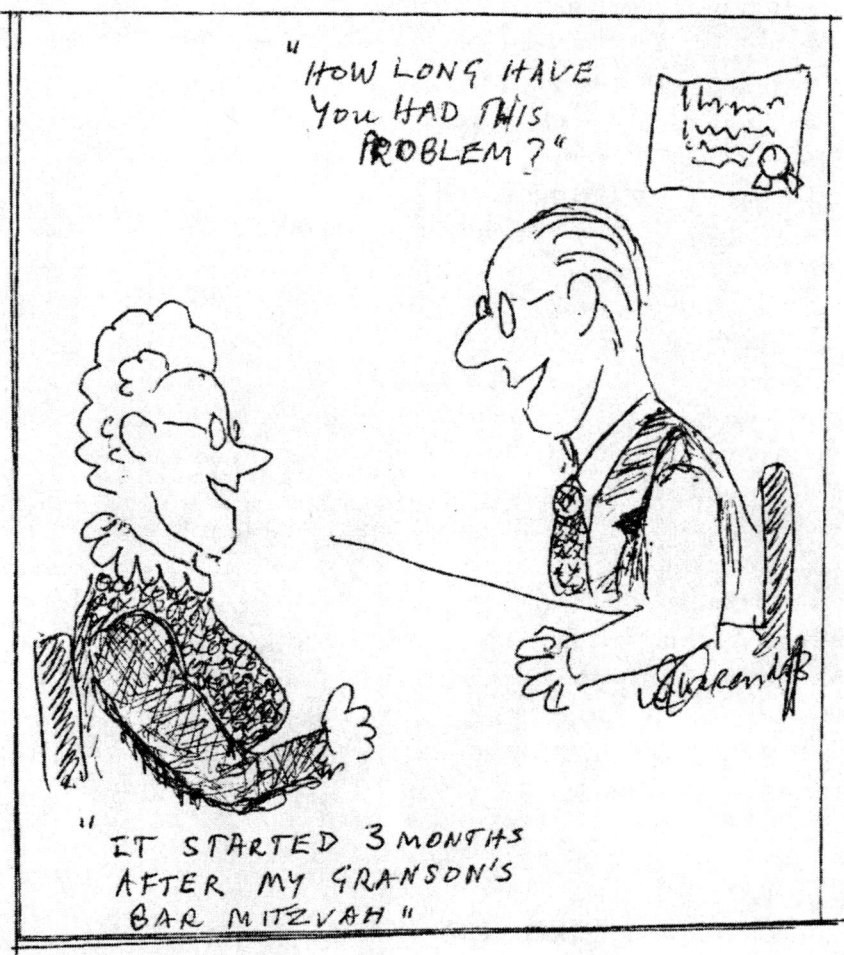

Getting the Point

All information obtained from the patient during history taking is extremely important.

This patient was a young man 32 years of age. He was employed in a sedentary job. He presented with severe sharp, stabbing pain which started in his hip and spread all the way down to the back of his thigh, calf and toes. His symptoms were typical of sciatica. He had been to several other specialists. He denied any history of injury and insisted the onset was spontaneous, several months prior. He described the pain as being constant and unrelieved by resting or any other measures that he had attempted.

The X-rays of his lumbar spine were normal. The neurological examination of his legs was normal. The examination of his back was normal and I have very little in the way of significant findings to go on. He was exquisitely tender in his right buttock and I arranged for X-rays of his pelvis and hips.

Lo and behold! Guess what?

To my amazement and considerable gratification the films reveal that there was a 2 ½" needle imbedded in the tissues of his buttock in the proximity to the sciatic nerve.

I showed the patient the needle and asked him how it got there. He was totally puzzled! He finally did recall that a few months ago when he came home from work his wife was sewing. Her supplies were arranged on the bed. He remembered that he had a "roll" with his wife on the bed. Shortly thereafter his "sciatica" began.

I subsequently carried out surgery and explored for the needle which was sticking into the sciatic nerve. The needle was removed and the patient made a complete recovery.

Snap Diagnosis

It is sometimes tempting, when the situation seems simple, to make a quick diagnosis without having all the facts and a complete history. Occasionally this can prove awkward and embarrassing.

In the earlier years of my practice, a gentleman presented with chronic pain in his shoulder. He said the pain was present all night and that he doesn't sleep.

"You mean the pain is so bad that it keeps you awake all night?" He replied, "No doctor, I am a night watchman."
So much for a snap diagnosis.

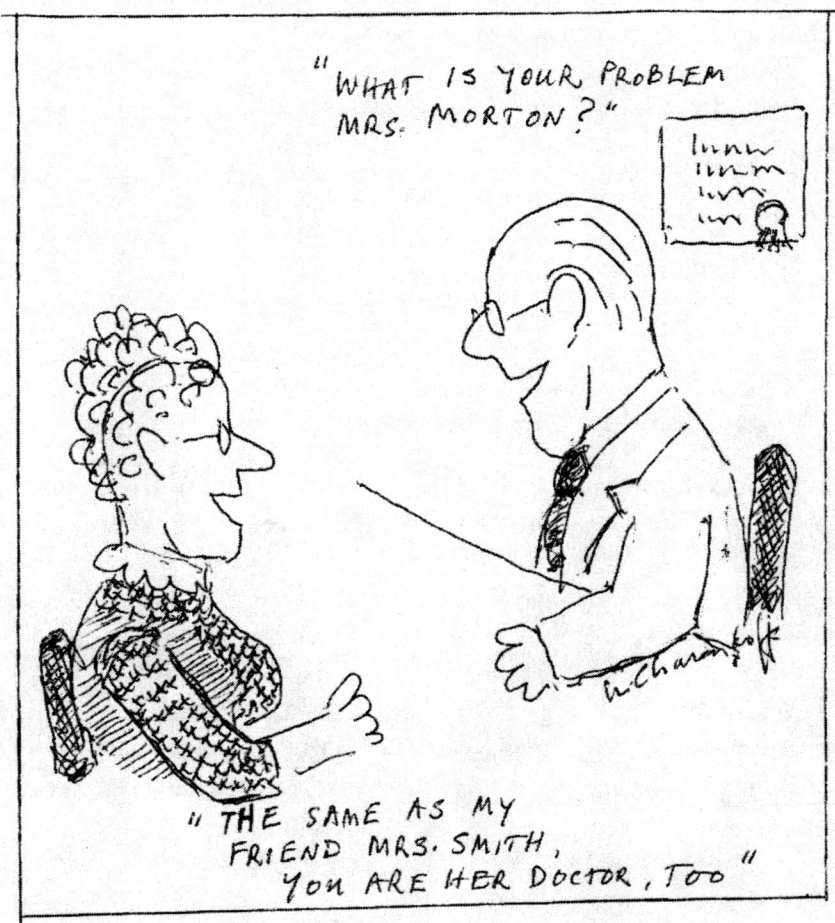

A Serial Operation

My patient was a middle-aged Jewish lady who spoke broken English. She presented with a back problem.

During the examination I noted that she had a lower abdominal scar and asked her to explain.

"Vell Dr. Charendoff I had woman's problem and my doctor a very big *(by which she meant a very important)* doctor is doing for me a very serial *(by which she meant serious)* operation."

She continued, "He is doing for me a hysterectum (by which she meant hysterectomy). He is also telling me I had trouble with mine "gentleman's entrance" (by which she meant genital) and he fixed that too."

Unusual Source of Referral

You never know where your next patient is coming from. One day on the golf course I was proceeding down a cart path when the golf cart behind me began to pick up speed. Apparently its brakes had failed. We were on a steep incline. The golf cart, with its two passengers, sped past me and did a cartwheel at the base of the hill landing upside down in the creek with both passengers pinned underneath.

A number of golfers had witnessed the accident and a rescue party was immediately organized. We went into the creek, freed the two golfers and pulled them up onto the bank. Fortunately they were still alive.

An ambulance was summoned. The two victims were taken to the hospital, where I was on staff.

I acquired two new patients that day.

"If I laugh at anything it is that I may not weep."
~ Byron ~

The Price and Power of Fame

"The best sense of humor belongs to the person who can laugh at himself."
~ anonymous ~

Aren't you...?

I had been on the active surgical staff at the North York Branson Hospital for many years, but had not had the occasion to visit for some time. One day I was requested to return and carry out a consultation.

Afterwards, I settled at the nursing station writing up my notes. There was also a nurse there, at the other end of the station. As I looked up from time to time to gather my thoughts, I noticed she was staring at me. Each time I caught her eye, she would look away as though embarrassed.

She finally apparently got up her confidence and approached me. She said, "Excuse me sir you look very familiar to me."

I said, "I was thinking the same when I saw you. You look familiar to me as well. Why do you ask?"

She said, "Didn't you used to be Dr. Charendoff?"

MEDICAL MIRTHOLOGY *(Finding Humor in Medical Practice)*

You are the Most Famous Doctor in Canada

The patient was a middle-aged gentleman. He had been referred to me from the United States for an orthopaedic consultation. He greeted me with the words, "Dr. Charendoff, you must be the most famous doctor in Canada."

I modestly asked why. He answered, "From my home state, I called the long distance operator, and asked for the phone number of Dr. M. Charendoff. Without needing to look it up, the operator immediately gave me your phone number."

I must admit I was surprised myself. However, I later found out the operator happened to be a patient of mine, and had my phone number memorized.

Unexpected Celebrity

It was our first trip to Israel. My wife and I wanted to visit the Hadassah University Hospital which was the location of the famous Chagall windows in Ein Karem. There are 12 windows which depict the 12 tribes of Israel and Jacob blessing his sons.

When we arrived it was apparent that an important function was in progress. The area was completely cordoned off to hold back the throngs of visitors. There was security everywhere. Each exit was guarded by an armed Israeli soldier. There was no way we were going to get in.

I decided to approach one of the guards to explain we were visiting from Canada and would be disappointed if we did not have the opportunity to visit and view the windows. "Excuse me," I said hopefully. "My name is Dr. Charendoff..."

To my surprise he did not even allow me to complete the sentence.

"Dr. Charendoff, go right in. We have been expecting you." With that he brushed aside a number of the tourists and cleared a path for myself and my wife. He opened the door and allowed us into the Synagogue. He then resumed his position outside.

Inside, the chapel was overflowing with guests but we were able to find two seats. We wondered what the soldier meant when he said they had been expecting us. How did he know we were going to be there that morning, when we ourselves didn't know until that very day?

I asked the gentleman beside me if he could fill me in, and then everything made sense.

We were about to witness a briss, a ritual circumcision. The father was a professor of medicine at the university and the whole Department of Medicine had been invited to the ceremony. The Israeli soldier upon hearing "Dr. Charendoff" must have assumed I was a member of the faculty and an invited guest.

After the briss I introduced myself to the new father and offered congratulations. I apologized for being there under false pretences. He thought the whole episode was extremely amusing and graciously invited my wife and myself to stay on for the refreshments!

The moral of this story? It's not who you know, but who they think you are.

The Portrait

One of my hobbies is painting, and a few years ago I was requested to do the cover portrait for a publication called Canadian Doctor.

Dr. Bean, whose portrait I was to do, lived in western part of the country and I was in Toronto. So I arranged for him to send me his photographs as obviously sitting for his portrait personally was out of the question.

When I completed the portrait it was duly published and I donated it to Dr. Bean.

A few years later I was attending a meeting at the University of

Toronto dealing with post-graduate training of interns. At that time I was chairman of the program at the North York Branson Hospital. As I entered the committee room, I immediately recognized Dr. Bean from the photographs he has sent.

He had moved to Toronto and was now serving on the same committee. He had never met me personally.

I went over to him and without introducing myself asked how he liked his portrait. He was rather puzzled and taken aback. "How did I know about it?"

After a few more leading questions I finally introduced myself. "I am Dr. Charendoff. The artist who did your portrait."

He then greeted me very warmly and thanked me profusely. He had loved the painting.

The Doctor Knows Best

My patient was an affluent businessman. I had operated upon his knee. We had become good friends. He was planning a business trip to England and Europe and invited me and my wife to join him and his wife as their guests.

He had contacts in London and Belgium. Everything was planned out to the last detail. We were picked up by a private uniformed chauffeur at Heathrow and driven to our hotel. We checked into a beautiful suite at the Dorchester in London. During our stay everything was provided for us – dinners and entertainment, first class restaurants, stage shows, private gambling clubs and the always-available chauffeur.

My wife and I discussed our good fortune and wondered how we could repay my patient for his kindness.

I noticed my friend was limping, and he explained his knee was giving him trouble. When we checked in at the airport my friend told me he was going to request a bulkhead seat so he could stretch his legs and be more comfortable on the return flight.

I watched as he limped to the check-in counter and spoke to the clerk. I noticed he was becoming more and more agitated as she shook her head. He returned to our group quite dejected.

In an attempt to reciprocate for everything he had done on this trip, I offered to request the bulkhead seats on medical grounds. After all, I was his orthopaedic surgeon and he was my patient.

Having nothing to lose I went to the check-in clerk.

"I am Dr. Charendoff. That gentleman over there who just spoke to you is my patient. He is having a problem with his knee and requires some consideration. Can you do anything for him?" The clerk explained there were no bulkhead seats available, and asked if he was well enough to fly.

I said he was, and was asked to return to the waiting lounge. The clerk would do what she could.

Our flight was called. As we were proceeding through the gate the purser looked at my ticket and said "are you Dr. Charendoff? And the other three are they in your party? Is your patient fit to travel?"

Again I said he was, and we were asked to step aside while the rest of the passengers boarded.

At this point my patient became furious at me. "Morris, they think I'm too sick to fly. I should not have listened to you and you should not have interfered!"

I thought perhaps he was right.

When all the passengers had boarded the purser came to me and said, "Dr. Charendoff I am sorry for this delay and I apologize for not having any bulkhead seats. The only thing I can offer you are four first class seats. No extra charge of course. I hope that's acceptable."

My friend had overheard this conversation and was dumbfounded. He offered a meek "thank you."

A Clash with the Law

I was driving home from the golf club on a beautiful bright summer afternoon. I felt very relaxed and started to daydream in anticipation of how I would spend the rest of the day. The road ahead was downhill. As I was approaching an underpass the speed limit was 45 mph and I inadvertently increased my speed to 55 mph as I proceeded under the bridge. Before I knew it there was a police officer waving me to the side of the road. He had parked his cruiser at the bottom of the hill and set up a radar surveillance. It was an excellent location to trap speeding drivers at the foot of the hill.

He approached my car. "Sir do you know how fast you were going?"

I was quite aware and did not attempt to offer any excuses or pleas for clemency. I simply pleaded guilty.

"Sir your driver's license please." I handed it over to him.

He looked at it and said, "So you are Dr. Charendoff?"

"Yes. Give me the ticket so I can go home."

"You are Dr. Charendoff, the orthopaedic surgeon?"

"Yes. Give me the ticket."

The officer broke into a broad smile. "Doc, no way am I giving you a ticket. Two years ago you did surgery on mother-in-law's feet. Before that she drove everybody crazy complaining about her painful feet. Since the operation she has been so happy there hasn't been a peep out of her."

Still Working

I am frequently asked at this stage in my life if I am still practicing. I always reply, "Yes, and I will continue to do so until I get perfect."

My 15 Minutes of Fame

During my surgical residency at the Jewish General Hospital in the late 40's, my chief had occasion to carry out abdominal surgery on a Mr. B.

In that era there was a famous exotic dancer performing in Montreal. Her name was Lily St. Cyr, and her performances were always sold out.

A day or so after Mr. B's surgery a call came over the intercom. "Dr. Charendoff there is a Lily St. Cyr at the nurse's station. She wants to talk to you."

Of course everyone in the hospital heard the same call. It turned out Mr. B was Lily St. Cyr's husband and she was inquiring about his condition.

Over the next few days she came in to visit her husband and each time the same call came over the intercom. "Dr. Charendoff, Lily St. Cyr to see you."

I was the envy of all the interns.

Instant Celebrity

A colleague called my office to say he was referring a patient for a second opinion.

"His name is Glen Gould. You will find him eccentric."

Already internationally recognized for his genious, Mr. Gould had sustained an injury to his neck and arm while abroad and was claiming it was impeding his performance.

When he came in I understood what his family physician had meant by "eccentric." On the day of our appointment Toronto was in the throws of a heat wave, yet he was wearing a winter cap, an overcoat, gloves and boots.

MEDICAL MIRTHOLOGY *(Finding Humor in Medical Practice)*

I took his history and we proceeded into the examining room.

I said, "Please take off your clothing for the examination." He removed his outer clothing consisting of the overcoat, scarf, gloves, two sweaters, shirt and undershirt. He was sweating profusely and felt clammy. Although he removed his shirt he kept it draped over his shoulders and back. He removed his boots and I noted he was wearing a pair of heavy socks.

After the examination he quickly got dressed. I reassured him about his orthopaedic status and said I would send the report to his doctor.

Glen Gould attributed his problem to an incident when someone as a friendly gesture slapped him on the back. He was suing for damages resulting from the injury. During his travels he had consulted numerous specialists in the United States, Europe and Canada. The consultation with me was much more than a "second opinion."

He continued to perform brilliantly as far as the critics were concerned, but insisted his performances were not up to his standards.

In his book "Glen Gould as patient" by Peter Oswald, MD, states "he feared he might never be able to play the piano again and that his career was ruined. He asked his lawyer to take action against Steinways for $300,000 in personal damages. ... On February 4, 1960 he was seen by Dr. Morris D. Charendoff, one of Toronto's leading orthopaedic surgeons. ... What Dr. Charendoff concluded was (Glen) could have suffered a minor traction injury to the various nerves entering the upper extremities (neuropraxia). They can usually last anywhere from 6 to 8 weeks, but do not lead to permanent disability."

Peter Oswald continues "By the summer of 1960 Gould was already back to giving concerts and making recordings and films."

Lost and Found

When my son Jay was 5 years old he wandered away from home with his little friend and ended up on the runway of Downsview Airport, several miles away. All air traffic was halted while the two wanderers were picked up by a security vehicle and brought into the terminal control room. Of course the children did not have any ID. In response to questioning my son said, "My name is Jay Charendoff. My father is an orthopaedic sturgeon at the Mount Cyanide Hospital."

The security officer was then able to locate me and arrangements were made to return the two young explorers to their respective homes.

Have We Met Before?

An Italian patient brought her 19-year-old son with her to the office to act as a translator. As I was conversant in Italian I didn't request assistance. When I finally finished the consultation the patient said to her son, "Tell Dr. Charendoff I am angry at him."

I was surprised by her comment and asked why.

"Because you didn't recognize him. When my son was a newborn you treated him for his club feet for more than one year." I had not seen him since then. The mother was right. I didn't recognize him. However his feet were quite straight and she was happy about that.

MEDICAL MIRTHOLOGY (*Finding Humor in Medical Practice*)

Everything is Relative

"Humor is like a needle and thread. Deftly used, it can patch up just about everything."
~ *anonymous* ~

Adventures with My Colleagues

"Doctors are men who prescribe medicines of which they know little, to cure diseases of which they know less, in human beings of whom they know nothing."
~ Voltaire ~

The Irish Orderly

When I was interning at the Jewish General Hospital in Montreal there was an Irish orderly who had been working that capacity for about 25 years. He was extremely professional and well regarded by all. He also had a good sense of humour.

His favourite expression was, "I'm Irish, you know. I have taken more shit from Jews than any other Irishman in the world."

The Volunteer

In medical school when we reach the "the clinical years," we get exposure to actual patients. The class of 150 students were divided into small groups and assigned a clinician teacher.

On this particular day our group was to have an instructional clinic on the performance of a lumbar puncture. We were gathered in the treatment room. The nurse wheeled in the patient and placed him on a table. He was positioned facing the wall with his knees curled up and with his back to our group.

The clinician explained the technique to us, while the nurse prepped the patient.

"Has anyone ever done a lumbar puncture?"

"No."

"Has anyone ever seen a lumbar puncture?"

"No."

"Would anyone like to volunteer to do one now?"

The group as a whole backed off nervously and declined, not wanting to be embarrassed.

Except one.

This fellow had an abrasive, aggressive and obnoxious personality, and was quite pushy. He was told by the clinician to scrub and put on his rubber gloves. The clinician made it clear it was important to keep the patient informed as to what was happening, especially since he was facing the wall.

The volunteer armed himself with a 6-inch needle, approached the patient's back and then, remembering the clinician's caution, said to the patient, "Sir, you are going to feel a little prick at your back."

Truer words were never spoken.

My Secretaries

About a year after I went into practice and when I could afford it, I hired my first medical secretary. I asked whether she had plans for the future which might interfere with her job, and she said no.

Within a few months however she became engaged, got married and became pregnant. In due course she had to quit working, but said to me "I have a cousin about my age and she is also a medical secretary."

I hired her, after inquiring as to her long-term plans. Within a few months she also became engaged, got married and became pregnant. She had to quit work as well.

The word got out if you want to get pregnant, work for Dr. Charendoff.

Special Instruments

One particular operating room nurse I was working with had a reputation for being cocky and arrogant. She would never admit a mistake.

In orthopaedic surgery we use many specialized instruments, such as periosteal elevators, nerve elevators and a variety of retractors.

During the course of one operation I asked the scrub nurse for an "Otis elevator." She did not have one, but requested it from the know-it-all, who promptly offered to get it. After a search of the instrument room she returned rather flustered. I explained she would find the elevator in the hall. "You know the instrument which is used to take people up and down from one floor to another?"

She blushed.

I later fooled her again when I requested a "fallopian tube."

Doctors Are Not Infallible

A doctor friend of mine went to his country club. He was an avid swimmer and was preparing to go into the pool. Now in the locker room, he was called to the phone. He spoke briefly to his office, and then put on his bathing cap and donned his bathrobe. He proceeded to the pool, removed his robe and dove into the beckoning water.

There was one slight problem. He had been distracted by the phone call and had forgotten to put on his bathing suit.

Splash!

Good Enough to Eat

My wife and I were out for dinner with another couple. During the meal my friend's hearing aid started acting up, so he decided to remove it and place it on his bread and butter plate.

He proceeded to order escargot and during the dinner he placed the shells on the same plate.

At the conclusion of the dinner he reached for his hearing aid. It had been cleared along with the shells.

He confronted the waiter. "Where are the escargot shells?"

The waiter took him to the kitchen and showed him a large garbage bag filled with hundreds of shells.

"There," he said.

My embarrassed friend had to sift through the shells, all of which resembled his hearing aid.

He finally did find the elusive device. Or was it really a shell he put back in his ear?

"Live and Learn"

Live and Learn

During his orthopaedic rotation I asked the intern about the patient with a knee problem. "What does IDK mean?" (In orthopaedics it means internal derangement of the knee.)

"I don't know," he replied.

Another intern was in the habit of putting GOK for the provisional diagnosis. I asked him what he meant.

"God only knows."

"A man reallly isn't poor, if he can still laugh."
~ anonymous ~

Medical School (Mis)Adventures

"A medical degree is no substitute for clairvoyance."
~ George Bernard Shaw ~

Blood Money

When I was doing my postgraduate training interns were not paid. The Red Cross would pay $25 for each blood donation and I became a regular donor to supplement my income.

This blood money helped me and my wife survive.

Close Call

When I applied to medical school at the University of Toronto, there were 650 applications for the program but the government insisted only 150 of the best applicants be selected in order to ensure there would be very little chance of failure. The government needed doctors to serve in the Armed Forces, as World War II was on at the time.

If a student failed first year, he could not repeat and was automatically drafted into the Armed Forces. The competition accordingly was very intense.

At the conclusion of the first year final examinations the results were on the bulletin board of the medical school building. On the appointed day we gathered anxiously to check the results. When my turn came I checked the list under the heading PASS.

My name was not there!

I felt crushed and couldn't understand, because I was a good student. My world had dissolved and my future plans disintegrated. On my way home I wondered where I went wrong. What would I tell my parents? This meant the end of my medical career and induction into the Army.

On my way home I met several of my classmates. They proceeded to congratulate me! I didn't know what they were talking about. "What do you mean? My name wasn't under the pass list."

They explained there was another list marked "Passed with Honours." I ran back to the medical school and sure enough that's where my name was after all.

After it finally hit me I had passed with honours in my first year of medical school, I could finally laugh at myself and my mistake.

New Edition

My medical school class and many others before and after had a fantastic professor of anatomy, Dr. J. C. Boileau Grant. In the middle of our course the eagerly awaited new edition of his "Grant's Anatomy" was published.

It was much sought after by medical students and teachers alike. I read it cover to cover. One particular anatomical diagram caught my attention.

Could I be wrong or was this an error? It appeared to me that the organs were transposed. I read and re-read the text and reviewed the diagram to confirm my suspicion and I concluded it was indeed an error.

What to do? I brought this to the attention of some of my classmates. The consensus was I should forget it and not get involved.

But I couldn't and I did. I determined to point out the error to Professor Grant.

I timidly made an appointment to meet with him, and arrived in his office with my copy of "Grant's Atlas of Anatomy" under my arm.

He greeted me in a most pleasant and gracious manner. Yes Mr. Charendoff, what can I do for you?"

"Professor Grant, I may be wrong but I believe there is an error in your new edition which I would like to point out to you. Sir."

I turned to the page and to the diagram. My heart was in my mouth. What if I was wrong?

He studied the diagram for a moment and said "You are quite right. The organs are transposed. Quite right Mr. Charendoff."

He was very appreciative and extremely pleased with me. He continued, "I will have this error corrected by the publisher."

I was elated! He even offered me a job as demonstrator in the Department of Anatomy.

I got an A on my final examination!

On-Call and Ready

During my internship rotation I was on call in the emergency department. After a particularly busy session I finally went to the doctor's call room to get some sleep.

A ringing phone woke me up. The nurse explained there was a patient in the emergency department and I was needed.

"OK. I'm on my way" I mumbled, half asleep.

Tired as I was I got up and went to the emergency room. Then the phone rang again and I heard the nurse's voice asking, "Where are you, we are waiting!"

I blinked strongly, and realized after the first call I had fallen asleep again and just dreamt I had gone to the emergency department.

MEDICAL MIRTHOLOGY (*Finding Humor in Medical Practice*)

You're in the Army

When I enrolled in medical school World War II was on. All first year students were automatically enlisted in the Canadian Officers Training Corps.

Company R, our class, was the medical division. We were obliged to spend two weeks at a training camp in Niagara-on-the-Lake and were to be transported there by ship from Toronto.

On the appointed day all students assembled in full battle dress at the docks at the foot of Bay Street to board the S.S. Cayuga.

I explained this to my parents, but they were concerned I maybe wasn't telling the whole story. They suspected something else was going on, and the sight of me leaving the house in full battle dress and carrying a rifle was most alarming.

As I boarded the S.S. Cayuga I caught sight of them on the docks. They had come to see me off thinking I was being shipped overseas.

Funny Bone

The funny bone is located at the elbow, and if you bang it on something you will feel nerve shocks and pins and needles spreading into your fingers.

Why is it called the "funny bone?"

As one of my professors of anatomy explained, it is because of its location on the "humerus" (arm bone).

The Quota

When I graduated from medical school I wanted to specialize in orthopaedic surgery and had to get a residency position. In Toronto at the time, there was a wonderful surgical training program called The Gallie Course. My academic record was excellent and I was well qualified.

The only problem was I was Jewish and felt my chances of being accepted there were non-existent. Accordingly I accepted a residency training program in Montreal at the Royal Victoria Hospital instead.

After spending 5 years there my chief, who was a wonderful teacher and human being, asked me about my future plans. I told him I wanted to take some further training in trauma surgery specifically at the Department of Veteran's Affairs Hospital in Toronto (now Sunnybrook). I also added it was impossible for me to get into the Gallie Course because I was Jewish.

He was stunned. "I know Dr. Harris, currently the professor of surgery there. If you wish I will give him a call."

I was thrilled.

A few days later I was told the position was mine.

Where the Gallie Course had previously been closed to me, it was suddenly made available by a simple phone call. I did complete my training at the University of Toronto, and was probably the only Jewish resident to do so at that time.

The Waiting Game

Here's another story where it's easier to laugh about it afterwards.

When I finished my post-graduate training in orthopaedic surgery I was one of 14 candidates in Canada qualified to sit for the written examinations. Only seven of the initial applicants were successful and were permitted to take the oral examinations. I was one of them.

These oral examinations took place over a 2-day period, and at their conclusion the group gathered in a waiting room to be informed of the results.

MEDICAL MIRTHOLOGY (*Finding Humor in Medical Practice*)

After waiting for about one hour the door opened and a secretary entered. She read off four names and asked these candidates to come with her, leaving three of us remaining in the waiting room. We obviously did not know which group had been successful.

A few moments later the door opened once again and the secretary entered. "You three doctors have nothing to worry about."

"A sense of humor can help you overlook the unattractive, tolerate the unpleasant, cope with the unexpected and smile through the unbearable."

~ anonymous ~

Hospitals

"Medicine is the only profession that labors incessantly to destroy the reason for its own existence."
~ James Joyce ~

Hospital Call

I was doing a pathology residency at the Jewish General Hospital in Montreal. The chief pathologist was Dr. Simon and his technician was Monsieur Legault, responsible for maintaining the morgue and preparing the bodies for autopsy. Monsieur Legault was an excellent technician.

One day an autopsy was scheduled. Dr. Simon and I went to the autopsy room. The body was on the table covered with a sheet. Everything appeared to be in order, however Monsieur Legault could not be located. In spite of several calls to switchboard there was no sign of him. Dr. Simon was becoming more and more irritated and eventually he said "I don't know where the hell Legault is, but we will start without him."

He removed the sheet from the body and there lying on the autopsy table was our own Monsieur Legault. He had taken a few drinks, lay down on the autopsy table, covered himself with a sheet and then had a fatal heart attack.

He had prepared himself quite well.

My Mexican Interns

When I was chair of the Intern Training and Education Committee at the North York Branson Hospital we accepted 6 graduates from the University of Mexico. These Interns were very dedicated and a pleasure to train.

Being somewhat fluent in Spanish and wishing to improve my language skills further, I made an arrangement with them. When they rotated through my service on orthopaedics they would speak only Spanish to me I to them.

This applied not only to orthopaedic rounds and patient teaching, but also during surgical procedures.

They all agreed and it worked out well.

As a result I was likely the only Jewish orthopaedic surgeon in Canada who operated in Spanish.

"Muchas Gracias!"

Every Little Bit Helps

I was doing a surgical residency at the Royal Victoria Hospital in Montreal. A middle-aged Jewish lady was scheduled to undergo an abdominal operation (laparotomy) to establish a diagnosis of her gastrointestinal complaints.

With advanced technology today a laparoscopy would probably be done through a small incision, but in those days the abdomen had to be opened up. The anaesthetic of choice was a spinal block during which the patient was also sedated, but not unconscious.

The operation proceeded uneventfully. The surgeon examined each organ and nonchalantly enumerated the condition of each organ in turn. "The esophagus and stomach appear normal. The duodenum appears normal. The gallbladder and bile duct appeared normal."

When he had completed his enumeration the patient, who was obviously paying attention more than we realized, suddenly spoke up in her sedated state to make sure nothing had been overlooked. "You didn't mention one thing. How's my liver?"

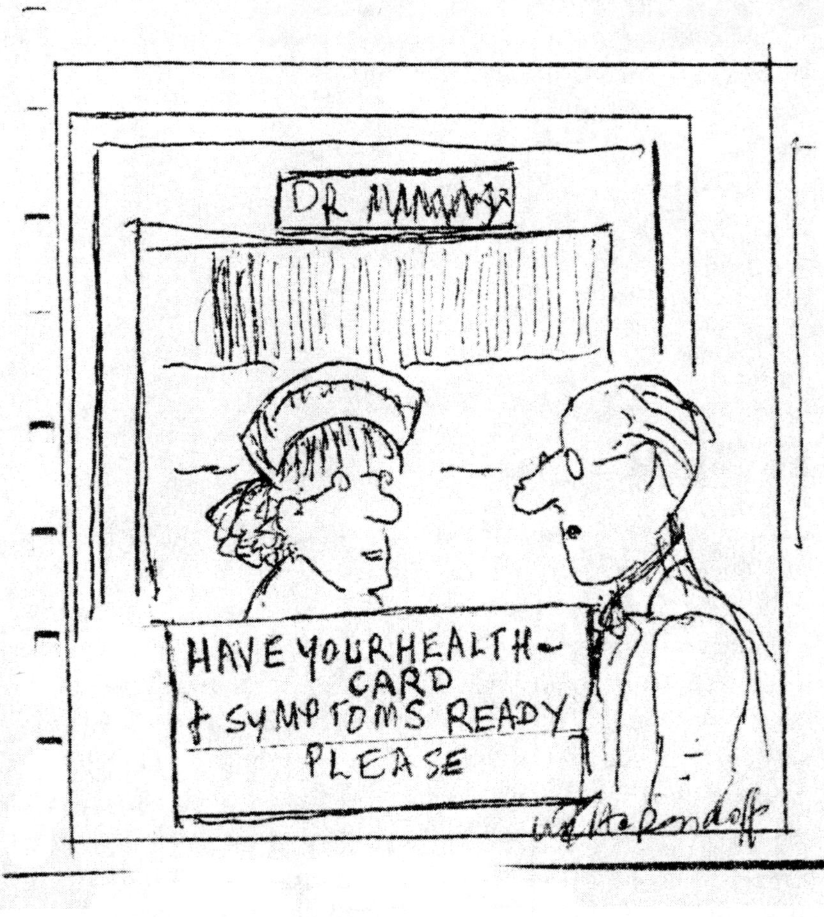

The Power of Prayer

I was invited to join the staff of the North York Branson Hospital, a facility administered by the 7th Day Adventist Church. I was about to perform my first surgical procedure, but was not yet too familiar with their policies.

Just before the surgery my assistant, a 7th Day Adventist physician, said "Dr. Charendoff, before you scrub come into the operating room with me."

The patient was on the table, but not yet under anaesthetic. My assistant took the patient's hand and my hand and knelt down to pray finishing with, "Dear Lord please steady Dr. Charendoff's hand."

The surgery continued uneventfully, but I was not certain if the prayer was a regular preoperative custom, or whether my reputation had preceded me.

Chinese Food

In Montreal there was an extremely popular Chinese restaurant called Ruby Foos. On my intern's pittance I could not afford to take my wife there. However when we had visitors from Toronto we were always taken to Ruby Foos.

On this particular occasion I was on call at the hospital. The restaurant was only 10 minutes away. I told switchboard where I was going to be, and left the phone number of the restaurant with instructions for the operator to call me if necessary. I was not disappearing, I was following custom and letting her know how to reach me.

Sure enough halfway through dinner the waiter approached our table and said, "Dr. Charendoff, there is a call for you."

"Hello," I said. "This is Dr. Charendoff."

To my surprise and horror, the voice on the other end said "This is Dr. Kaufman." My knees almost buckled. Here was the Chief of Surgery himself calling me! Instead of phoning me directly, the operator must have given him my contact number. He continued, "I am at the hospital. I need you here now."

Although there was no harm done I was rather embarassed by the experience. Over the next 24 hours we performed 14 appendectomies —a hospital record.

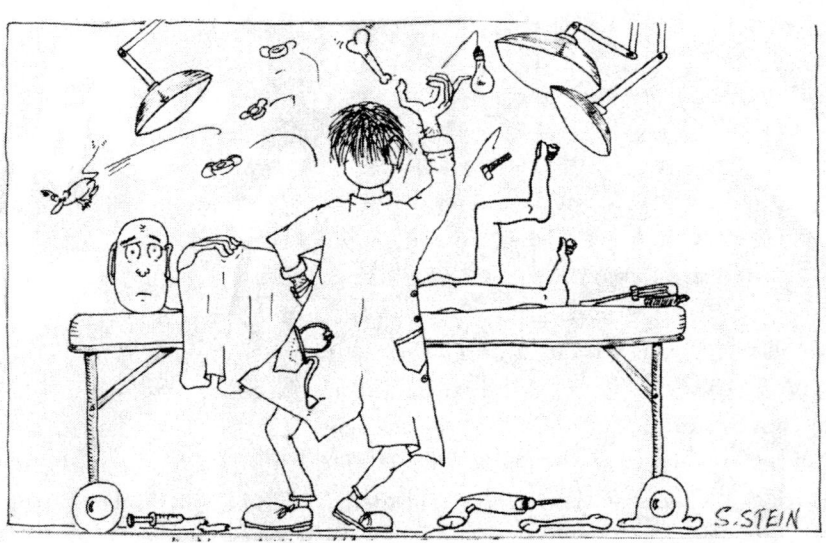

"You will have to stop eating all that junk food!"

The Long and the Short

Patients come in different shapes and sizes. On occasion their physical dimensions can pose problems. I remember two such individuals.

The first was a gentleman about 6' 8" tall. He could not fit comfortably into a hospital bed unless he curled up in the fetal position. We arranged to place another bed at the foot of his, so he could stretch his legs.

The other patient was a young man who weighed 275 lb. He was scheduled for spine surgery. It was impossible to place him on the regular operating room table without him rolling off to one side or the other. Accordingly we had to place two operating tables side by side to accommodate his bulk.

Egg Rolls?

An Orthodox Jewish patient of mine was operated on for a fractured hip. Postoperatively the nurse reported to me she was refusing to eat, and after several days they were becoming concerned.

I called her son and suggested he visit his mother to find out if there was some favorite food that perhaps would lure her to eat again. He did so and to his amazement found she was asking for egg rolls.

As his mother was Orthodox, he did not understand. This Chinese delicacy is not Kosher as it contains pork.

The son however got the requested egg rolls and brought them to his mother. She saw them and exclaimed, "This is traif!" (Traif means non-Kosher.)

She brushed the food aside and again stated. "I vant egg rolls."

It subsequently was determined she was constipated and was asking for the laxative "Agerol."

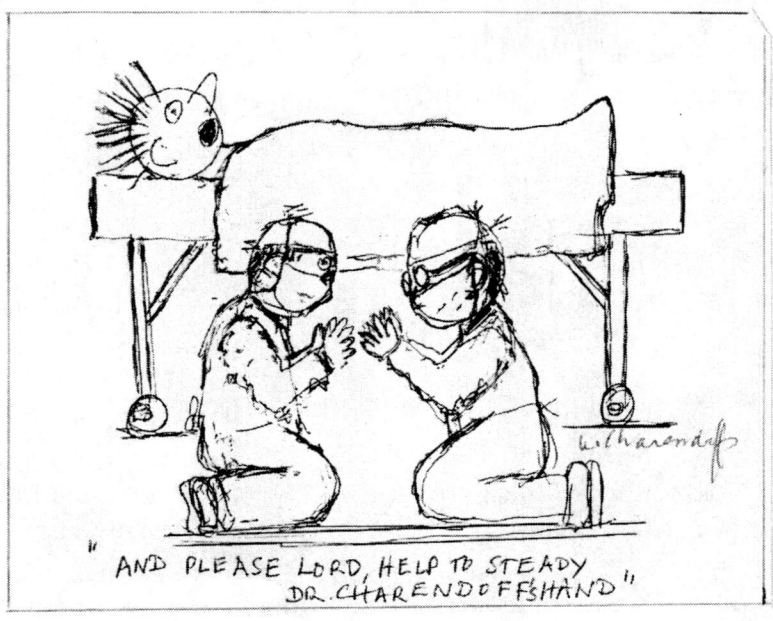

"AND PLEASE LORD, HELP TO STEADY DR. CHARENDOFF'S HAND"

The Complete Job

When I was training there was a pathologist at the hospital named Dr. Simon. Of course he also carried out the autopsies.

The in joke at the hospital was:
    1. The patient was admitted.
    2. The patient was diagnosed.
    3. The patient was treated.
    4. The patient expired.
    5. The patient was Simonized.

Yuletide

One Christmas I had two patients in a semi-private room. Their beds were side by side. One patient was Mrs. Lamb and the other was Mrs. Sheppard.

The Intern

I was once performing an operation with the assistance of a junior intern, who was unfortunately completely inept. His could not follow simple instructions, and his assistance was more of a hindrance. We were all getting frustrated.

Aware he was annoying every one, the intern said, "Dr. Charendoff tell me what to do." To which I replied, "Go into psychiatry."

Bed Shortage

All hospitals experience bed shortages. Over the years various policies have been devised to make better use of the available beds.

I once suggested to the administrator of our hospital we could double the patient capacity without any expensive renovations. He asked me how.

"Currently we have semi-private rooms, meaning two patients to each room. Why not change the designation of semi-private and have two patients to each bed?"

The administrator said he'd think about it.

MORRIS D. CHARENDOFF

"A desire to take medicine is perhaps the great feature which distinguishes man from other animals."
~ Sir William Osler ~

MEDICAL MIRTHOLOGY (*Finding Humor in Medical Practice*)

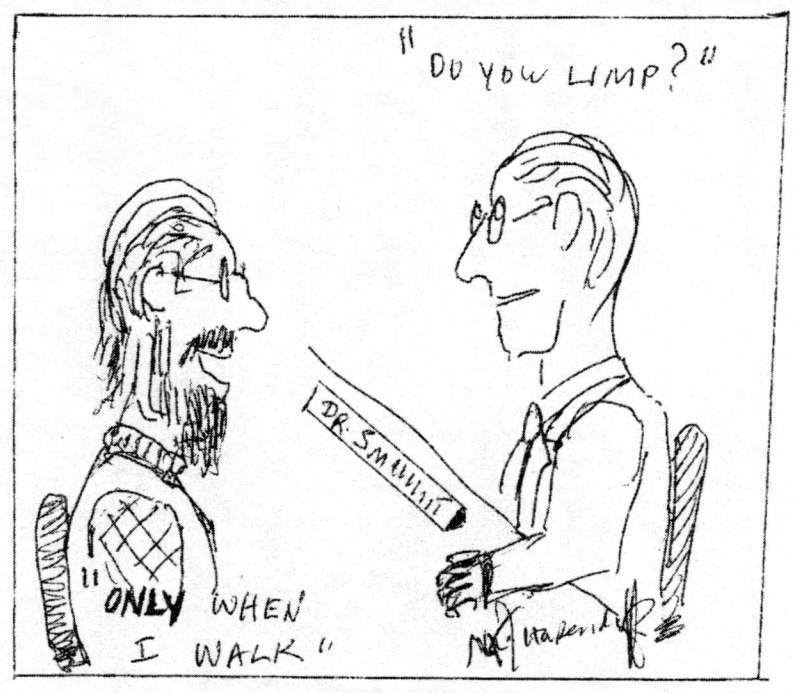

Patients, Patient or Otherwise

"A good laugh is the best medicine, whether you are sick or not."
~ anonymous ~

As you sew so shall you reap

The gentleman was a patient of mine with whom I was well acquainted. He was referred to me for pain and swelling involving the sole of his foot.

He informed me about one year earlier, while at his cottage, he was walking barefoot on the wooden dock. He slipped and got a 1-inch sliver in his foot. He went to the hospital in the country and had it removed, however his foot did not recover.

When I examined him it was apparent he still had a foreign body in his foot, which was causing the pain, limping and swelling. I suggested surgery and he agreed.

At the operation I removed a 2-inch piece of the wooden pier left in his foot and this "sliver" measured about the thickness of a pencil. It had been there for a whole year.

As I knew him well enough I decided to have some fun with it.

I placed the "specimen" in a test tube together with some flowers I obtained from another patient, and left the test tube at his bedside. At rounds the next morning I explained to him the sliver in his foot had been there for so long it had taken root and bloomed, hence the flowers.

At first he was not sure if I was serious, but then he accepted the whole episode in good humor.

MEDICAL MIRTHOLOGY (*Finding Humor in Medical Practice*)

Squeaky Joint

A young man came into the emergency department with a knee injury. During the examination, each time I flexed and extended his knee there was a rather audible squeak.

He asked, "What's wrong doctor? Why is my knee squeaking like that?"

He was reassured when I explained to him that it wasn't his knee squeaking, it was the stretcher.

The Private Patient

Before the days of government-subsidized medical services, patients paid for their own doctor's fees. Some patients could not, and so most hospitals had out-patient clinics where they received care at no charge.

These clinics were staffed by family physicians and specialists in all fields of expertise. All doctors on the hospital staff were obliged to donate some of their time to care for these "clinic patients." They did so gladly as a service to the community.

Patients received the same care from the doctors whether their status was "clinic" or "private." The system worked well, but occasionally a clinic patient felt stigmatized by the arrangement and aspired to upgrade to private status.

One such lady appeared in my office one day. I recognized her from having attended her at the clinic.

"Hello Mrs. G. How are you? Why are you here instead of at the clinic?"

"I want to be your private patient."

I knew her financial circumstances and said, "You realize it's not necessary. You will get the same treatment from me at the clinic, but here as a private patient I will have to charge you."

"I know, but I want to be your private patient."

She had very bad bunions and painful feet. I told her she could be helped by an operation and she agreed.

After the successful, uneventful operation I sent her a bill for $100. About 3 months later she returned to the office for a check up.

In her broken English, she said, "Dr. Charendoff, denk you for the operation. You have goldina hands. I am very happy wit my new feets."

She reached into her purse and extracted my bill.

"I want to talk to you about your bill. I know it is very fair, but $100.00 is a lot of money for me. I would appreciate it if you could make a discount."

"Certainly. What would make you happy?"

"Maybe you can take off $25."

I took the bill and crossed off the $100.00 and wrote balance $75. She replaced my bill in her purse. About a month later she returned to my office, full of complimentary remarks.

She again removed the discounted bill and said, "You are a vunderful doctor and so kind, but you know $75 is a lot for me."

"I understand. What will make you happy."

"Maybe you can take $25 off."

I discounted the bill again for her, and she again replaced it in her purse.

The same scenario repeated itself on subsequent visits, until the balance was zero dollars. In her mind she believed that she had paid my bill.

On the final visit she blessed me up and down. "Thank you for treating me as a private patient. When it comes to my health money is no object. I told my friends about you and I will be sending you lots of patients – just like me!"

MEDICAL MIRTHOLOGY (*Finding Humor in Medical Practice*)

The important patient

I arrived at the office quite late. I was on call in the emergency department at Branson Hospital and had been treating a lot of trauma patients that day. My receptionist had explained this to the patients in the waiting room, which by now was overflowing.

Most patients accepted the situation graciously and with resignation.

One unhappy gentleman was ushered into the exam room when his turn came, by which time I was about 1-1/2 hours behind schedule. I apologized for the delay but he was quite indignant and hostile.

"That's not good enough Dr. Charendoff. I am a very important businessman. You have kept me waiting too long. My time is very important."

My apology fell on deaf ears.

In due course he was billed for the consultation. My invoice was returned unpaid with the following note: "Dr. Charendoff I am not paying your bill. You kept me waiting for 1-1/2 hours. I am a very important man. My time is worth $200/hour. You owe me $300 and I expect to be paid."

I discussed the situation with some of my colleagues and friends. My goals were to get paid for my services and to retain his goodwill if possible. I was not going to pay his bill.

The situation was a problem in public relations.

I wrote to him, "I am returning your bill unpaid. I am certain your time is worth $200/hour as you said and had I sought your services I would gladly pay. However I didn't. You sought mine. You were under no compulsion to wait for 1-1/2 hours, and could have left and rebooked. The reason for the delay was explained and I apologized. I expect you to pay my bill."

In due course he did pay my bill and gratefully thanked me for having helped him with his orthopaedic problem. It later came to my attention his business failed and he went into bankruptcy.

I felt sorry for him, but felt certain his failure had nothing to do with having waited in my office.

Two to Tango

One day a young construction worker came to the office with a foot problem. I said to him, "Take off your boots and socks. I'll be back in a minute."

When I returned I saw he had removed only the boot and sock of the foot giving him trouble. I examined it and said, "Now take off the other boot and sock."

His face reddened visibly. He did so reluctantly, and I soon understood why. The good foot was filthy and grimy.

He had not anticipated I'd need to examine both feet, and had washed only the foot giving him trouble.

Chiropractic Care

A lovely young woman about 40 years of age presented with severe sciatica and neurological problems involving her legs. She had not responded to physiotherapy. It was her first visit to my office. She felt she was getting progressively worse and more disabled.

Following the examination and review of her X-rays, I told her she would probably require back surgery. Of course she was reluctant.

She wanted to see her chiropractor first. She told me he was a Dr. Hull.

I chuckled to myself and said, "It might be of interest to you to know

Dr. Hull is currently a patient in the Branson Hospital orthopaedic floor, room 302. I just did back surgery on him a few days ago for severe sciatica. If you want to go to him first, that is where you will find him.

Without further discussion she replied, "Dr. Charendoff book me for the operation."

Grateful Patients

I have a sign in my office waiting room which reads: "Everyone brings joy to this office. Some when they enter, some when they leave."

I have been extremely fortunate in my practice in that, proportionately, the first group outnumbers the second by a ratio of 99:1, and probably more.

In my experience, most patients are genuine, compliant and extremely grateful, and are forever desirous of showing this appreciation for the caring interest, understanding and kindness extended to them.

My practice consists of a very diverse ethnic mix. Each group tends to demonstrate goodwill in its own unique fashion, but the common denominator is their generosity. I am sure most doctors have been recipients of tokens of appreciation and various gifts on occasions from their patients.

Most of these items are usually brought during holiday season, such as Christmas, New Year's and Hanukkah, and similar special occasions. At these times my office becomes a veritable cornucopia. My family and staff also become the beneficiaries.

But my good fortune does not appear to be confined only to those special times. Three examples of patients come to mind.

Example 1:

One patient, a very fine Portuguese auto mechanic, never fails to call the office a few days prior to his scheduled appointment. He usually starts with, "I will be there on Monday at 11 a.m. for my appointment. How many staff will be there?"

"Six. Why?"

He then brings in lunch for eight consisting of foods such as barbecued chicken, rice, potatoes and dessert, all of which are fabulous. My offer to pay him is always greeted by a wave of his hand and a benign smile. He has been repeating the same pattern for many years. My office staff always eagerly awaits his next appointment. His arrival brings us joy. And no, we don't call him the chicken man.

Example 2:

I had two patients, a husband and wife, who were plagued by back problems. I subsequently performed spinal surgery on each one about two years apart. They were extremely pleased with their results. They remained patients for other problems for many years.

One summer evening, my wife and I were having a barbecue for our whole family. We were all gathered on the deck. Unannounced these two patients arrived at the house carrying a little bundle wrapped in a blanket and said, "Dr. C, we have something for you."

The "something" turned out to be a six-week-old Boston Bull Terrier. My family fell in love immediately with the beautiful dog, whom we named Poppi. The dog has been in our family for many years and represents one of the most heartfelt tokens of appreciation I have ever received. She is a member of our family. She has brought joy to all who have come to know her and is a constant reminder of those thoughtful patients.

MEDICAL MIRTHOLOGY (*Finding Humor in Medical Practice*)

Example 3:

The patient was the wife of an Italian cabinet maker, and they were both recent immigrants to Canada. She presented at my office with what turned out to be an extremely serious knee problem and subsequently required arthrodesis of the knee. She was about 40 years of age at the time. Her husband expressed concern about the costs involved, explaining he could not afford the operation as he had just started to work in this country. I told him not to worry, as that under the circumstances, there would be no charge for my services. The operation was successful. The patient was eventually discharged from my care and I more or less lost track of her.

About a year later, I received a phone call at home. It was the patient's husband. "Dr. C. I have something for you. I'd like to bring it to your house."

When he arrived at my house, I thanked him for his gift and suggested he place it on the kitchen counter.

"You don't understand. It's something which I made and it will not sit on the kitchen counter."

He had brought two men with him to assist him. They unloaded the article from the back of a truck and carried it into the dining room. It was a dining room server about a metre and a half long, French provincial in style. It was a most beautiful creation!

He told me that for one year, he had worked evenings and weekends on his own time at the furniture factory where he was employed. He had designed and built the buffet by himself. He and his helpers brought it into the dining room where it has stood for many years. I was truly amazed. He would accept no payment and just said, "You saved Maria's life."

MORRIS D. CHARENDOFF

House Calls

When I first started practice it was not unusual for doctors to make house calls, even specialists.

I received a call from a doctor, saying a patient of his was totally incapacitated with severe back pain and was not responding to any treatment. Would I make a house call?

I agreed, and when I arrived at the house I found a middle-aged obese gentleman. He was lying on his back on the living room floor in agony. He was sweating profusely, and his wife was hovering about helplessly. He had been lying there for 24 hours refusing to be touched or moved. He could hardly answer my questions, but kept repeating, "It's my back! it's my back!"

I had to lie down beside him to try to get some history. Apparently his pain started a day earlier when he bent over and the severe attack persisted. None of the medications ordered by his physician had helped.

I told him I would have to turn him over to check his back. Screaming with pain he reluctantly agreed and kept repeating, "Don't hurt me."

I took his shoulders and hips and started to roll him onto his side like a log, trying to be as gentle as possible. About half way to my goal I heard a loud CRACK, like dry wood breaking. His wife also heard it and paled perceptively. I had no idea what was happening.

The patient suddenly bellowed, "Doctor it's gone. The pain is gone!"

He jumped to his feet and started running around the room with a very happy broad smile like a carved pumpkin. He kept repeating, "I'm cured. You are a fantastic doctor."

Everyone was happy and I was the most relieved of all. I never did establish a diagnosis, but I believe that he had a subluxation of one of his lumbar facet joints which inadvertently reduced itself as I was rolling him over.

MEDICAL MIRTHOLOGY (*Finding Humor in Medical Practice*)

Another House Call?

I was called by a family physician who informed me he had a patient with a dislocated shoulder and he wanted me to take care of it.

I had completed my orthopaedic training and was in practice for only a short time. I was used to treating trauma patients in the emergency department of a hospital. Accordingly I asked, "OK what hospital is he in?"

"He is not in a hospital. He is lying between 2nd and 3rd base on the baseball field in Bellwood's Park. I want you to treat him there. I'll meet you."

When I arrived there was a group of baseball players gathered around the patient who was lying in the dirt at about the shortstop position. He had made the play, but had fallen. His shoulder was obviously dislocated and his arm was in a grotesque position. He was in agony.

I lay down in the dirt beside him. I took off my shoe and placed my foot in his armpit. I told the family physician to give him Demerol. I applied traction to his arm and shortly thereafter his shoulder joint snapped back into position with an audible and satisfying thud.

In a moment or two the patient jumped to his feet and began testing his arm movements.

Feeling no pain he exclaimed, "OK, let's play ball!"

He was quite disappointed when I told him he would have to wear a sling for 3 weeks.

The Tree Surgeon

I was called to the emergency room to attend to a young man with a fractured leg. He was employed as a tree surgeon (pruning, removing dead limbs, etc). He told me he had fallen out of a tree from a height of about 10 to 12 feet. I subsequently reported the accident to the Worker's

Compensation Board as follows. "Dear Sir, Mr. A. sustained a fracture of his tibia when he fell out of his patient."

WCB acknowledged the accident, but the humorous aspect made no apparent impact.

Where there is a will...

I had occasion to operate upon a young lady about 35 years of age. She had a back problem for which she required spinal surgery. She was recovering nicely and all was going well.

About the third day postoperatively, while I was making rounds, the curtain was drawn around her bed. There were signs of "activity" going on and I was aware of some noises from behind the curtain.

I asked the nurse what was happening. She told me that the patient had a visitor, her husband. He eventually appeared from behind the curtain.

He said, "Dr. Charendoff I would like to talk to you when you when you have finished checking my wife."

"Okay, I will meet you in the hall."

The patient was fine. In the hallway the husband asked, "Dr. Charendoff how long after this surgery is permissible to resume... You know... Do you know what I mean?"

I told him I got his meaning and said, "It depends. Is your wife in a private or semi-private room?"

He said she was in a semi-private room, but I don't think that deterred him.

You Can't Be Too Careful

An 85 year old lady was brought to the emergency room. She had fallen and a fractured hip was suspected. X-rays were ordered, but she adamantly refused to have them. She explained, "I heard if I have too many X-rays it could be harmful to the grandchildren!"

A Jamaican lady with a chest problem presented in emergency. She was asked if she had ever been X-rayed. She replied, "not only have I been X-rayed, but I have been ultraviolated!"

Compliant Patient

The postoperative patient was instructed not to get his dressing wet. When he appeared at the office for a check up one week later his dressing was loose and in disarray.

When asked why he said, "I did what you told me. I took the dressing off each time I had a shower."

The Baby

I had occasion to operate upon a 75-year-old gentleman who had sustained a fractured hip. Postoperatively he did well. One day as he was making rounds the nursing supervisor on the ward told me one of the patient's relatives was visiting and wanted to talk to me. The relative had the same surname as the patient.

As I approached there was an elderly gentleman pacing up and down in the corridor outside the room.

He came up to me and asked "Are you Dr. Charendoff? I am Mr. A (the same name as the patient)."

I immediately concluded that he was the patient's brother.

"You made an operation on him. I am his father. Tell me how is my baby?"

I was totally amazed. I guess one never stops worrying about one's children.

Postoperative Complication

I had an Italian gentleman 65 years of age who had chronic low back pain. He had undergone back surgery elsewhere and subsequently consulted me.

He kept coming back to me postoperatively explaining he had a complication which had rendered him impotent and ruined his sex life. He wanted to sue the doctor who did the surgery explaining, "He cut the nerve to my peanuts!"

Insult to Injury

I was called to examine a patient brought in following a skiing accident. I was not prepared for what I found.

There lying on a stretcher was a young woman still in her ski outfit. Both her legs were in splints from the toes to about the knees. I recognized her immediately as she was a friend of the family.

"What happened to you Ruth? I didn't know you were a skier."

"I'm not. This is the first time I have been on skis."

I imagined that she had gone down a steep hill and had fallen. Something spectacular, certainly.

"Tell me about it."

"I was taking my first lesson. The instructor had me start at the beginner's slope, a very slight incline only about 2 feet high. As I took my first step and pushed off, my skis crossed and I fell so here I am. I never want to ski again."

She had fractured both ankles. Fortunately she made a good recovery. Indeed she had had enough of skiing and never went again.

A Miraculous Recovery

A few years after I had been in practice an acquaintance of mine called.

"Morris," he said, "I would like you to look after my father. He has a fractured hip." I said I would be happy to do so, and to make the arrangements.

The son continued, "I have to fill you in on my father's background. He has been in a mental institution for 25 years. During that time he has not spoken or recognized anyone in the family. He is not violent. The doctors do not know the exact diagnosis. He fell in the mental institution yesterday. He has been X-rayed there and has a fractured hip."

I said, "Fine. Bring him to Mount Sinai together with his X-rays."

In due course I carried out surgery on his hip. I visited him in the recovery room to check on his condition. He was already awake. "Mr. G., how do you feel?" I asked not expecting a response.

To my amazement he replied "I'm fine. Are you the doctor who operated upon me?" I was stunned. I called his son and said "I thought your father hasn't spoken in 25 years?"

"That's right he hasn't."

"Well he is speaking now and he is quite lucid."

The son came to the hospital and was flabbergasted. He had a long conversation with his father, the first in many, many years. There was no indication of his mental illness. As far as the son was concerned, his father was back to normal.

"Morris what did you do?"

"I operated on his hip."

My colleague's father was able to leave the institution and return home. No further sign of mental ilness developed.

Professional Wrestler

I once had as a patient a professional wrestler. He had been injured in an accident. He was a gentleman about 40 years of age and had an amazing physique. He weighed about 275 lb. His muscles were huge.

He pointed out where his pain was located and as I touched the affected spot he suddenly bellowed with pain and dropped to his knees.

He screamed, "That's it! That's it, I give up!"

It was the first time I had wrestled a professional wrestler. Although I did not pin him, I did drop him to his knees.

MEDICAL MIRTHOLOGY *(Finding Humor in Medical Practice)*

Cast-Aways and Cast-Offs

When a patient is treated for a fracture the very presence of the cast appears to attract a variety of foreign objects. Frequently the patient experiences itchiness or similar discomfort under the cast and finds a number of unique methods of relieving the unpleasant sensations.

I have discovered a number of such items when the cast is finally removed. A partial list includes:
1. Toothbrushes.
2. Knitting needles.
3. Pennies.
4. Pieces of coat hangers.

It is not unusual for such items to be trapped under the cast eventually resulting in a skin ulcer leading to infection and unpleasant odours.

Patients are frequently instructed not to get the cast wet. It is not unusual for them to remove it, take a shower and replace the dry cast thus following the doctor's instructions. On occasion the patient will disobey the doctor's orders and take a shower or bath with the cast on thus turning the cast into a useless, soggy bandage.

Furthermore if the patient feels the cast is too long and is irritating the arm or leg they go about trimming it until is completely useless in immobilizing the fracture or there is nothing more left of the cast.

"As it is not proper to cure the eyes without the head nor the head without the body so neither is it proper to cure the body without the soul."
~ Socrates ~

Medical Miscellanae

"Imagination was given to man to compensate for what he is not, and a sense of humor to console him for what he is."
~ anonymous ~

A technological world

We live in a world programmed with advancing technology, automatic answering machines and computers. If you phone any company chances are you will get an automatic voice which states, "Your call is very important to us. Please wait. A representative will be with you shortly."

Rarely do you get to speak with a human being. You are usually put on hold. The music begins and the message occasionally repeats itself.

I thought of applying this technique to my office.

"This is Dr. Charendoff's office. If you are calling about back pain press 1. If you are calling about shoulder pain press 2. If you are calling about knee pain press 3. Your call is important to us. Please stay on the line. A medical person will assist you shortly. Feel better."

Knee Reflexes

If you test knee reflexes while standing in front of the patient it could result in a kick to the groin and be hazardous to your health.

MEDICAL MIRTHOLOGY (*Finding Humor in Medical Practice*)

You Have to be a Golfer

A number of years ago I was playing golf with my usual foursome. It was in mid-October, and there was a slight drizzle. The paths were covered with leaves and were somewhat slippery. One of my playing partners was a heavy gentleman, who weighed about 275 lb. As we were walking to the next green he disappeared over a slight knoll. Suddenly I heard him calling, "Morris, Morris come quick! I broke my leg."

From the sound from his voice I knew he was serious. I ran to him as quickly as possible. He was grimacing with pain and said "It's my right ankle."

When I looked at his foot it was twisted around so badly his toes were practically facing backwards. I removed his golf shoe and his sock. His foot and ankle were distorted, dead white and pulseless. He had an obvious fracture dislocation of his ankle.

A small crowd of golfers had collected. I told one to contact the pro shop on the emergency phone and to call 911. I gave my friend a cold drink to sip on.

"I have to set your foot temporarily to restore the circulation. It's going to hurt."

He nodded his approval and told me to go ahead. I gave him a tee to bite on. I straightened his foot and was overjoyed to note it pinked up and the circulation returned right away.

Then I had to immobilize his injury, so I took two golf clubs and made a splint using a number of towels and whatever else was available. He was much more comfortable.

When the emergency golf cart had arrived, it took 6 of us to lift him onto the stretcher and transport him back to the club house. He was taken to the hospital where X-rays revealed a serious fracture dislocation of his ankle. He underwent surgery by a colleague of mine who was on call.

As you can image word quickly spread throughout the club about the incident and the role I had played in his initial treatment. Many of the members approached me to make inquiries. No one asked how the accident happened. No one asked what kind of surgery he had. No one asked how he was doing.

Most of the members who I spoke to said, "I understand that you had to provide emergency care and that you made a splint out of a golf club." I replied I had.

"What club did you use?"

Gut Feeling

I had never been to a camp before, having spent most of my summers working and earning money in preparation for the next school year.

But during my second year of surgical residency, I got a call from a friend who was a camp director. A new children's camp was about to open and he asked if I would be interested in setting up the infirmary. He asked me to prepare a complete medical program to take care of the campers, hire a nurse and purchase all the necessary supplies. If I agreed to do so, I would be spending one month at the camp in Huntsville, Ontario, with my wife and one-year-old son.

I agreed, and made arrangements for a short leave of absence from my residency. We arrived a few days prior to the campers and the nurse and I set up the infirmary. When the campers and their parents arrived, there was the usual assortment of problems including allergies and dietary restrictions.

Being surgically oriented, the one problem I dreaded most was missing an acute abdominal problem like an appendicitis and confusing it with stomachache, homesickness or just something the camper ate.

Late in the afternoon of the first day a 10-year-old girl was brought to the infirmary. She was complaining of a stomachache which had started a couple of hours earlier, coincidentally just after her parents left.

I checked her out. She appeared a bit flushed and was running a low-grade fever, but nothing else was unusual. I admitted her to the infirmary as a precaution and we continued to check her over and

MEDICAL MIRTHOLOGY (*Finding Humor in Medical Practice*)

monitor her for the next few hours. Her temperature began to go up, but she did not experience any nausea or vomiting. Toward the early evening, she began to display tenderness localized to the right lower quadrant. By 10:30 I was convinced she was suffering from an attack of acute appendicitis.

I contacted the camp director and told him, "This child will require surgery." I called her parents to explain the situation, and suggested we send her home to Toronto (app. three hours away) and her parents contact their surgeon to make the necessary arrangements. The other option would be to take her into the hospital in Huntsville, which was 45 minutes away, and have the surgeon on staff carry out the operation.

The father asked if it was safe to transport her to Toronto, considering the inevitable delays. I told him I was not sure. "We would like her to have the operation in Huntsville. However we do not know any of the doctors there, but we do know you and accordingly, we want you and no one else to do the operation."

Needless to say, I was stunned. Here I was about to take a patient to a hospital where I was not on staff and where I had no privileges and where I was not known. I explained to the camp director the anticipated problems with the hospital. However, I was not concerned about doing the operation as I had done it on many occasions.

The patient was loaded into a station wagon with the nurse and myself and the camp director.

Upon arriving n Huntsville, I presented myself to the admitting officer. "I am Dr. Charendoff. I have a patient with acute appendicitis. She will have to be admitted and will require an emergency appendectomy."

"You are not on staff, are you?"

"No."

""Then we will refer the patient to our surgeon."

"You don't understand, I have strict instructions from the parents that no one else is to do the operation except myself."

The admitting officer disappeared into an adjoining office where a long telephone conversation ensued.

"OK, Dr. Charendoff, you can admit the patient and we will make arrangements with the operating room."

At approximately midnight on the first day as a camp doctor, I carried out the emergency appendectomy. The patient did have advanced acute appendicitis, and her abdominal pain was not merely due to homesickness or something she had eaten.

The surgery and her recovery went uneventfully. After a few days she was sent back to Toronto to convalesce. The patient returned to camp about 10 days after the operation to complete her summer holiday. She was brought back by her grateful parents.

This was during the pre-medicare days, and they insisted I bill them for the surgery. It was the first fee I earned in private practice.

Courteous Professional

In the days before medicare, I had a patient who was the recent widow of a former colleague. I had known him casually, as he had referred patients to me for consultation. I did not know his wife.

When she was in the consultation room I expressed my condolences and continued with the examination. She was troubled with low back pain. Attempting to calm her apprehension over her back, I explained her problem was not serious.

She was quite pleased. She smiled and thanked me then added, "By the way, you extend professional courtesy to doctors and their families, don't you?"

It has always been my policy to extend professional courtesy to patients who are doctors and members of their families, however remote. What I found annoying was she found it necessary to bring it to my attention as I would have offered this courtesy anyway.

In my most diplomatic manner, I assured her she need not be concerned, that "professional courtesy" would be extended to her under the circumstances and it had been my pleasure to take care of her.

About two years later, I noted on my appointment list a woman's name I was unfamiliar with. However, when she was ushered in, it turned out to be the same patient – the doctor's widow. She had developed a further orthopaedic problem. I was pleased she was apparently satisfied with my previous management of her low back pain and had no hesitation returning to my care.

I suddenly remembered our previous encounter and found myself thinking, "Aha! Back again!" As it was apparent she had remarried, I further said to myself this time, there would be no professional courtesy.

I offered my congratulations on her remarriage and we proceeded with her new complaint – bunions, as I recall but that is incidental to the story. I explained the treatment she required. Again she thanked me profusely and then...

"By the way, doctor, I know you practise 'professional courtesy.'"

"That's right," I said. "I extend professional courtesy to doctors, members of their family, nurses, men of the cloth..."

Before I could finish, she broke in, "That's wonderful and very kind of you. My second husband is a clergyman!"

Foiled again!

Sometimes you can't win. In spite of the above incident, I still practise professional courtesy. I feel honoured to take care of physicians, their families (even widows of doctors) and men of the cloth.

It is a rewarding and gratifying experience to know your colleagues have faith in submitting themselves to your care.

Been There. Done That.

The patient was a 25 year old girl with a back problem. After taking the history I instructed her to remove her outer clothing and put on an examining gown. I left the room stating I would be back with a nurse.

When we returned the patient was standing there stark naked. I tried to keep a straight face as she said, "Let's get on with it doctor. You've seen it all before."

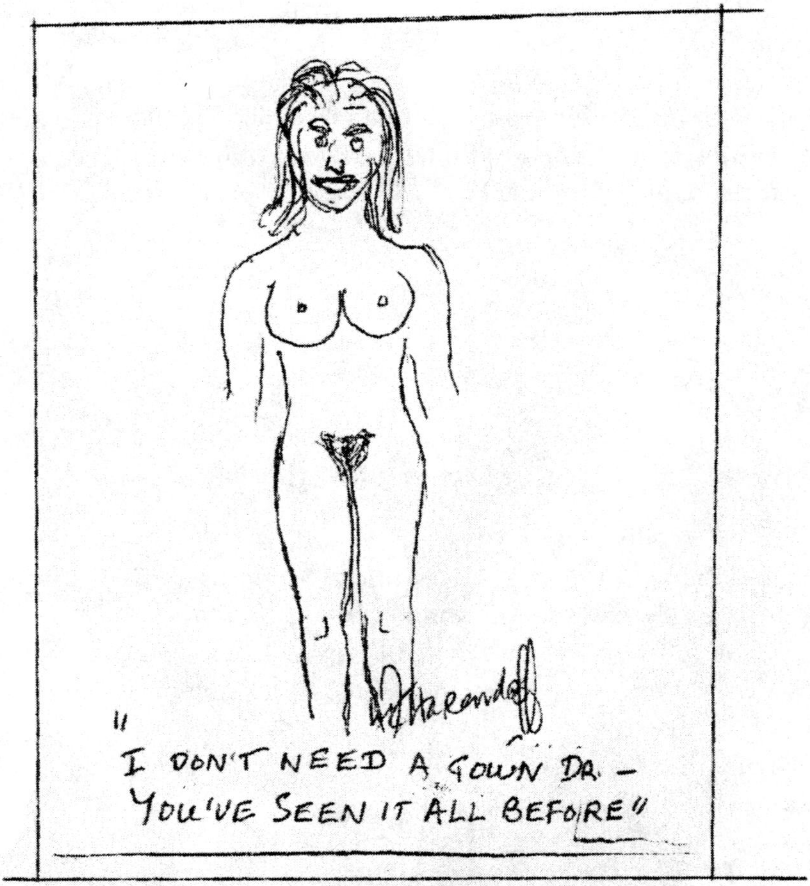

The Age of Specialization

You may ask what is the difference between a consultant and a specialist. Let me illustrate as follows.

I used to have a pet cat. He would stay all night roaming the neighborhood and spreading good will. Many cats were the recipient of his favours. The problem however was he kept the whole neighborhood awake with his wailing, and I received numerous complaints.

I finally decided to have "Tom" castrated. Now he still goes at night, but only in the capacity of a consultant.

General Practitioner Vis-a-vis Specialist

Is there is a difference? Judge for yourself.

A G.P. is a doctor who knows a little bit about a lot of things. A specialist is a doctor who knows a lot about a little bit.

As times goes on and with more information available, a G.P knows less and less about more where as a specialist knows more and more about less.

Finally the G.P. knows nothing about everything and the specialist knows everything about nothing.

Our 1st Car

After World War II it was extremely difficult to buy a car, as new cars were being manufactured slowly and the demand was great.

However, in 1947 we were finally able to get a Studebaker convertible. It had a black exterior and red leather interior. All our friends were envious. After 500 miles a first inspection was required and when the time came I left the car with the dealer for the weekend.

At 2:30 a.m. my phone rang. This was not unusual as I was on call. However the call was very unusual.

"Is this Dr. Charendoff?" Ths is Sargeant McTavish of the police department.

"Yes," I said anxiously.

"Do you have a black Studebaker convertible you left at the dealership?"

"Yes," I answered more anxiously than before.

"Doctor, your car has been stolen and we think it has been used in a hold up as a getaway car."

The car had indeed been used in a hold up and it was a few days before it was recovered. There was no damage, but it was no longer black. It was covered with white powder both outside and inside. It had been dusted for fingerprints.

9 Lives – 8 More to Go

One of my secretaries had a pet cat that was hit by a car. The cat was reasonably unhurt except it was limping. I suggested she bring the cat into the office. When the cat was examined I noticed she was limping on her right hind leg. X-rays revealed a dislocation of the hip joint.

My secretary asked me to take care of it. My first such case in a series of one.

We devised a plan. The cat was coaxed to eat some food containing a sedative. One staff member was assigned to each of the cat's extremities and another to hold the cat's head. We all took up our positions.

I then carried out a reduction maneuver to set the dislocated hip.

After several attempts there was an audible satisfying click as the dislocated joint settled into position. The cat was still somewhat sedated, but almost immediately jumped and began running about the office. The limp was gone. X-rays confirmed that the "operation" had been successful.

The cat lived to enjoy her other 8 lives.

Smuggling

You may have heard of trichinosis, a disease caused by parasites present in pork products. Jewish dietary laws do not permit the consumption of pork for this reason.

On one of our trips to Florida, my wife and I packed a salami and some bagels, as little treats to munch on. As we were going through Customs at the Toronto airport a young gentile Customs official asked, "Are you carrying any pork products?"

I answered, "No."

He opened one of the bags and retrieved the salami. It was about 12 inches long with a string tied to one end. He dangled the salami in front of us, and accused us of attempting to smuggle a pork product into the United States.

I answered, "Do you read Hebrew?" I pointed to the word Kosher in Hebrew stamped on the side of the salami and continued, "This word Kosher means it does not contain any pork products – only beef."

The Customs office was rather taken aback. "As far as I,m concerned this is a pork sausage. I don't read Hebrew."

He explained to his superior (who happened to be Jewish) we were attempting to smuggle a pork product into the United States and he held up the disputed salami.

His superior immediately recognized the item was Kosher, and contained no pork products. He explained this to his colleague who in turn said to us "I am dropping the charges. Carry on with your trip to the United States."

A Puzzlement

My mother-in-law was very proud of me. She thought I knew everything and constantly questioned me about her various symptoms. She was disappointed when I was unable to offer her an answer to her problems, whether they involved headaches, backache, stomach symptoms, etc. She would say, "You're the doctor. You should know."

"You are right," I would say. "But the problem is you are ahead of your time. You have symptoms for which a disease has not as yet been discovered."

Emission Control

In this highly technological age there is a great deal of concern with regard to how to control a variety of emissions such as radiation, light, sound, waste, etc.

Family physicians have to deal with a variety of emissions as well such as flatus, burps, gags, spit, sneezes, wax, belly button fluff, barf, b.o., urine, feces and perfume.

Accordingly routine medical practice also has its hazards. Some are avoidable, some are humourous and all can make every day at the office a new challenge.

Confucious Say...

It has occasionally been commented I should change my last name of Charendoff to something more easily remembered by anglophonic ears. Whenever this is suggested to me, I ask if the questioner remembers the name "Confucious." When told yes, they do, I say "You may remember his saying 'Man who sit on hot coals, char-end-off.'" They remember my name after that.

"Genuine humor is always kindly and gracious. It points out the weakness of humanity but shows no contempt and leaves no sting."
~ *anonymous* ~

Afterlaughs

"Our five senses are incomplete without the sixth — a sense of humor."
~ anonymous ~

This is a collection of tales from colleagues and a variety of other sources. Although not from my own practice, these adventures were presented as authentic.

A surgeon opened his practice in a primarily Jewish location. He placed the following sign in his waiting room: "Your killah is my gedilah." (Translation: "your hernia is my pleasure.")

When he subsequently moved to another location, primarily gentile, he changed the sign to read "Your rupture is my rapture."

A farmer underwent external skeletal fixation for a fracture of his tibia where pins and a metal rod were applied to the outside of his leg to hold the fracture in place. He was discharged with the hardware in place, as is the usual procedure, and given a follow-up appointment to have the metal removed in 3 months.

Somehow there was a lack of communication and he was lost to follow-up.

He returned to the clinic 3 years later. "The leg works great doc. I have been busy with my farming work, but when do I get the hardware removed?"

MEDICAL MIRTHOLOGY (*Finding Humor in Medical Practice*)

A grandfather wanted to visit his grandson, a doctor, who had recently graduated and gone into practice. He wanted to check out his grandson's professionalism and skills.

On the day of the appointment he was ushered into the doctor's office and went through a complete physical examination including lab tests. He was extremely impressed. He was told to wait for the results. Eventually his grandson the doctor brought him back to the consultation room.

"Grandpa your chest X-ray is okay, your electrocardiogram is okay, your urine specimen shows the presence of sodium chloride, a few white blood cells, a few red blood cells and a trace of sugar and albumin."

The grandfather paled visibly and said, "Then I must be very sick."

The doctor asked, "Why do you say that?"

To which his grandfather replied, "Well, in the whole specimen you mean there is no urine?"

A gentleman was in hospital awaiting surgery. He was visited by the organ recovery representative and asked if he would consider donating his organs in the event he did not recover. "Let me think about it," the patient said.

The next day the representative back to inquire if he had come to a decision. "Yes I have. I will donate my hernia."

A paediatrician gave the mother a prescription for her child's earache. He instructed her to instill the drops three times a day. One week later the mother returned saying his earache is no better, but his bottom is very sore. The prescription had read, "Instill two drops in R ear tid."

A frantic mother called the emergency room. "My baby ate some ants." The doctor explained ants were not harmful, and she didn't have to bring in the baby.

"That's good," said the mother. "I gave him some ant poison to kill the ants."

The doctor advised her to bring in her child right away.

During a vaginal hysterectomy the junior assistant, who had partaken of curry and beer the night before, could no longer control himself, and flatulated in the OR. The surgeon sniffed the air and said, "I smell feces."

The Chief Resident said he did as well.

The surgeon said, "I must have perforated the bowel. This could be fatal. I will have to open her abdomen." The junior assistant was presented with an ethical dilemma. Should he confess or remain silent and allow the patient to undergo a further, painful operation.

He leaned forward and said to the surgeon, "I think it was the nurse."

A probee nurse mistakenly entered the doctors' change room in the OR suite, where the elderly Chief of Surgery, having completed his caseload, was dressing to go home. He was in his shorts with one leg in his trousers. The nurse was quite embarrassed and turned red as she dashed out into the corridor. The surgeon followed, hopping into the corridor on one leg. He called after her, "Young lady, there is no need to run away from me when I'm dressing. It is when I'm undressing that you should be concerned."

The patient was an 85-year-old widower. His family decided it was time to admit him to a residence where he could get proper care, but he was reluctant. His son said, "Pa I have checked out a few places. I found one I think you will like. Let's at least go and pay it a visit."

The patient was not happy, but agreed.

When they arrived at the facility the son said, "Pa, I'm just going into the office for a moment. You wait in the lobby."

Two attendants were duly assigned to wait with the father, one on either side of him. A few minutes later he started to lean to the left. The attendant, thinking he was losing his balance, straightened him back up. Mr. Goldstein then leaned to the right and the other attendant promptly straightened him up once again.

The son son returned and said, "Pa the rooms are beautiful. Would you like to have a look?"

Mr. Goldstein said defiantly, "I hate this place already. They won't even let me fart."

My patient was employed as a spray painter. He presented with purulent sinusitis and nasal discharge.

"What colour is your nasal mucous discharge?"

"It all depends on the colour of paint I used yesterday."

Doctor: Show me your tongue.
The patient complies.
Doctor: Now show me your teeth.
The patient proceeds to remove his dentures and hand them to the doctor.

A female patient was recovering from hip surgery. A nurse was giving her a sponge bath, and the patient was covered with only a sheet. The surgeon was making rounds and as he entered the room the patient enthusiastically and joyfully raised both legs exclaiming "look what I can do!" With this exercise she threw off the bed sheet. She was not wearing undergarments.

The surgeon blushed.

The nurse asked the patient what kind of juice she would like, as she had to take some pills. The patient seemed perplexed. The nurse repeated the question, "What kind of juice do you like?" The patient replied, "My dear I have dated only gentiles."

A family physician was requested to make a house call. He left his bag open while gathering a few medical items from home, then snapped it shut and went on his way. When he arrived at the patient's home, he opened his bag and reached in to retrieve his stethoscope.

After a few seconds an appalling stench reached his nostrils. For a moment he was completely at a loss as to its source until a look at his hand showed the cat had used his medical bag as a "scratch" box.

After her hysterectomy a patient was given the usual discharge instructions. That night she called the doctor wanting to know if her mother could visit.

"Any time. Why do you ask?"

"It says here in your instructions no relations until after your postop check up."

A husband rushed into the local emergency room shouting excitingly, "My wife is going to have her baby in the taxi!" The ER physician grabbed his bag, rushed out to the cab and lifted the lady's dress. He suddenly noticed that there were several cabs and he had gotten into the wrong one.

For a routine check up the doctor saw the child's first name was Urine pronounced Youreen. The doctor curiously asked how her child came by such a distinguished sounding name.

The woman explained, "My baby was born premature and had to stay in a special nursing ward. She was really sick and they didn't know if she would make it, but the nurses said they would pray for her. I hadn't picked a name, but one day I came in and saw the nurses had already given her one. There was a piece of paper on an incubator that said "please save urine.""

A 75-year-old woman in the hospital for investigation of longstanding abdominal discomfort kept herself cheerful by flirting shamelessly with the male staff. During yet another round of tests she said to one handsome young doctor, "I wonder if you came up to my room and spent the night with me would it help me recover?"

The doctor replied, "It probably would dear, but I doubt your insurance would cover it."

My secretary told me in advance this patient was coming in. She had fallen out of an ambulance. I imagined a woman sick enough to require transportation to hospital in an ambulance and somehow fell out. Surely she would arrive at my office in a wheelchair hustled in by several embarrassed ambulance attendants, but she arrived alone and her story was much different from what I had imagined.

Yes she had indeed fallen out of the ambulance and broken her arm in doing so, but the vehicle was already stopped at the local hospital emergency department at the time. She was merely a passenger during the ride, sitting beside her husband who was a heart patient and was in distress. She had missed a step while exiting the ambulance and had fallen while following him.

They both survived.

When my mother appears in our waiting room to visit my associate everything gets lively. Against my pleadings mum insists on telling the other patients who she is. She becomes an instant celebrity. My patients invariably tell my mom how wonderful I am and later have nice things to say about her.

Mother discusses their various health problems and has an opinion about any ailment. One patient even said he could probably leave without seeing me, as mother set his complaints in order.

On some days, however, my mother prefers to stay anonymous and functions as a waiting room spy...

"Whose patient are you?"
"For how many years?"
"Do you like his care?"
"Does he ever talk about his mother?"

Body piercing and tattoos have become commonplace. One young man had his penis tattooed, which when in the flaccid state revealed lettering that could not be interpreted. The physician asked him for an explanation.

"Well doc he said you will have to take my word for it, but when I have an erection my penis sends a message to my girlfriend."

The physician decided not to pursue his curiosity and changed the subject.

In some situations it is difficult to keep a straight face.

A doctor once asked a young girl if she was sexually active. The patient replied, "Not really. I usually just lie there."

A med student did his first lumbar puncture on me. As I was curled in a ball he stuck the needle in my back. I said, "Am I supposed to see it coming out of my belly button?"

He just about dropped his pants.

One busy doctor has a sign in his waiting room which reads "have your symptoms ready please."

A postoperative gastrointestinal patient was told he could not eat until he was able to pass gas. The next day on rounds he had a sign around his neck stating "will fart for food."

The patient was recovering from gastrointestinal surgery. The nurse informed him, "The doctor says you can't eat until you pass gas."

Shortly thereafter the nurse heard him pass a large amount of gas in the toilet and remarked, "That sounds good enough to eat."

The other patient's visitors misunderstood.

The floor secretary on the ward complained she was not getting her lab printouts. I told her she needed to answer the message on her computer terminal to start the printer. She had no idea what I was talking about, so in frustration I explained, "Pull up your message screen and look for the cursing flasher."

"What?"
"You know, the cursing flasher."
She giggled and I realized I had meant to say the flashing cursor.

The following personalized license plates have been noted:
    Urology Resident: PPMD2B
    Cardiologist: LUBDUB
    Allergist: SNEEZE
    Orthopaedic Surgeon and gentleman farmer: BACKACRES

The amputee wearing an artificial leg tells his doctor, "I need a new prostitute. The old has one worn out."

A good speech should have a good beginning and good ending and the two should be as close together as possible.

The guest speaker at a medical convention was introduced and came up to the podium. He placed his watch on the podium and asked the Master of Ceremonies how long he could speak for, to which the M.C. replied, "You can speak as long as you like. We are all leaving in 10 minutes."

Patient (on telephone to the nurse): I have been in bed with the doctor for two weeks and he doesn't do no good. If things don't improve I will have to send for another doctor.

A French doctor had a patient who was convinced he was possessed by the devil. The doctor called a priest and a surgeon and equipped himself with a bag containing a live bat. The patient was told it would take a small operation to cure him.

The priest offered a prayer, and the surgeon made a slight incision in the man's side. Just as the cut was made, the doctor let the bat fly crying, "Behold the devil is gone!"

The patient believed it and was "cured."

An 85-year-old lost his wife and found a much younger girlfriend, barely 73 years of age, who said "Sam, every intimate relationship between a man and a woman should include sex. Ask your doctor for those blue pills advertised on TV."

So he did. He was a cardiac patient, but was not on nitrates so the medication was safe. At the next appointment, 3 months later, he showed up alive but said the Viagra hadn't worked.

When the doctor told him he could try doubling the dose he said with a smile and a hand on my shoulder, "Doc no way I am taking that chance. She will have to be satisfied with a cuddle. I know I am."

A nurse in her first year of training was, with the aid of an orderly, to transfer a deceased patient to the morgue. Arriving at the morgue she discovered she did not have the key. She instructed the orderly to remain with the deceased (covered by a white sheet) while she went to the office for the key.

Upon her return the stretcher covered by the white sheet was there, but there was no sign of the orderly. Suddenly in the dimly lit corridor she heard some wailing noises, and the sheet began to rise. The nurse was terrified.

The orderly had laid down on the stretcher beside the deceased, and covered himself with the sheet. The prank left a real mark on the nurse.

Two patients arrive in the office at 2 o'clock. One is booked for 2:45 and the other at 3 o'clock. At 2:30 both leave because they could not wait any longer.

A patient was discharged from the doctor's practice for non-compliance. She came back 3 months later to have her passport signed.

A patient was noted hammering on the bathroom door stating desperately, "I got to go in there! I am under the influence of a laxative."

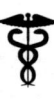

A wife was accompanying her ill husband who was being transported to hospital in an ambulance. She kept imploring the medics "Please take good care of him. I am dying that he should live."

George Burns was well into his 90's when his doctor advised him to eat only natural foods with no preservatives.

He replied, "At my age I need all the preservatives I can get."

Two psychologists met at their 20th college reunion. One of them looked quite old, worried and weathered. The other looked much younger.

The older one asked the other what's your secret. Listening to other people's problems for years on end has made me an old man. The younger looking one asked, "Who listens?"

The practice of medicine has changed over the years. Then again, it really hasn't.

Patient: "I have an earache."

Physician:

    2000 BC – Here, eat this root.

    1000 A.D. – That root is heathen. Say this prayer.

    1850 A.D. – That prayer is superstition. Drink this potion.

    1940 A.D. – That potion is snake oil. Swallow this pill.

    1985 A.D. – That pill is ineffective. Take this antibiotic.

    2000 A.D. – That antibiotic is artificial. Here, take this root.

MEDICAL MIRTHOLOGY (*Finding Humor in Medical Practice*)

A doctor had two female patients with opposite problems. One had a baby almost every year despite trying all kinds of birth devices. The other had been married 10 years and despite the use of fertility drugs she had no children. Both ladies happened to be named Liza. The doctor referred to them as "fertile-Liza" and "sterile-Liza."

There is a well-known song lyric reading, "The song is over, but the melody lingers on." To paraphrase, "the operation is over, but the malady lingers on."

A funny story can relax even the most anxious of parents-to-be. Try this one.

Jock and Heather lived in the remote highlands of Scotland. Heather was pregnant and about to go into labour.

Jock got on his horse and galloped 10 miles to fetch the doctor. When they returned it was in the middle of the night. The doctor told Jock to light the kerosene lamp as he made preparations.

In due course the baby was about to be born, and the doctor asked Jock to hold the lamp a little closer, which he did. He handed the baby off to Jock who wrapped it in a blanket and placed it into the cradle.

A few moments later the doctor said, "Jock, hold the lamp a little closer I feel something stirring." Another baby came along and again Jock wrapped the baby in a blanket and placed it in the cradle.

The doctor again said to Jock, "Hold the lamp a little closer, I feel something else is stirring."

At this point Jock became quite alarmed and said "Doctor you think it's the light that's attracting them?"

A lady brought her 10-year-old son to the doctor, as he was complaining of an earache. The doctor left the exam room open while the mother waited outside. The room was filled with a number of posters displaying anatomical parts of the body, communicable diseases, etc. The boy liked to read and focused on one of the posters. He read out loud: "When can I resume sex?" The mother quipped, "Just like his father."

My 60-year-old patient Mary was caregiver to both her parents, a very ill 85-year-old mother and a disabled 95-year-old father. Mary took Ma and Pa to a weekly bingo game. Ma was wheelchair bound would bark orders and clear a path with her cane. "Mary, move faster. Out of my way, someone will get our spot."

Once play started Ma quieted down. As the numbers were called Mary took a closer look at Ma across the table. Ma seemed to be falling forward. Her chest hit the table. She stayed there motionless. Mary ran to Ma and grabbed her and shook her shoulders, but there was no response so she screamed to call 911.

Now Bingo players are very intent on their game and they do not tolerate disturbances for long. So the caller droned on, "Under the O, 72. Under the B, 12." Ma's card was tended by a neighbour.

Just as the ambulance arrived, an old man who had been sitting beside Ma finished her card for her and yelled, "Bingo!"

MEDICAL MIRTHOLOGY (*Finding Humor in Medical Practice*)

I have always wondered how much of what you tell a patient he or she understands.

An obstetrical colleague reports his patient was newly married. She was 4 or 5 months pregnant and could not understand English very well. After the first examination, he gave her the usual prenatal instructions and hygienic advice and cautioned her not to go swimming.

The weather however was extremely hot. She disobeyed the doctor and went swimming in the lake.

At the next visit he prepared her for a possible cesarean section saying, "My dear you have a deficient passage. If you have a normal delivery it will be a miracle."

That evening the husband came home to find his young wife crying.
"What's wrong?"
"I went swimming against the doctor's order."
"And?"
"He told me I had de fish in de passage and if I have a normal delivery it will be a mackerel."

Two residents of a senior citizen facility became good friends. One was a widow and the other was a widower, and the question of marriage came up.

Neither was in really good health, so they decided to make some inquiries at the pharmacy.

Widower: Do you carry products such as heart pills, cholesterol pills, high blood pressure pills and diabetic medicine?

Pharmacist: Yes we do handle all of those products.

Widow: And do you also have hearing aids, canes, walkers, arthritis medicine and knee bandages?

Pharmacist: Yes we do handle all of the above products.

The couple then said to the pharmacist, "Good. We want to register here for our wedding gifts."

An elderly gentleman appeared at the fracture clinic. He brought with him his cast, which his wife had removed with a saw.

When asked why he had let his wife do this instead of having it done at the clinic, he replied, "We have been married for 60 years and I trust her implicitly, so I let her remove my cast. Why should I let you do it when I don't know you from Adam?"

Stressful situations can make you say strange things. A physiotherapist on a very busy psychiatric ward was once heard to state "My God this is a madhouse."

A doctor called the hospital and requested, "ICU." The operator responded, "I see you too."

Nurse to patient recovering from intestinal surgery: The doctor says you can have a clear liquid diet.
Patient: What does that mean?
Nurse: Anything you can see through.
Patient: In that case I'll have a dozen doughnuts.

MEDICAL MIRTHOLOGY (*Finding Humor in Medical Practice*)

The patient attended a gynecological clinic. She was positioned in a cubicle, prepared and draped. It was an extremely hot day and there was no air conditioning. The patient had an offensive odour emanating from her genitals, and the gynecologist had to hold his breath. The examining doctor started the pelvic examination, felt something and directed the patient to push. With that the patient flatulated.

The doctor turned to the nurse and said, "Thank God for a little fresh air."

Dictated – roseola infantum
Transcribed – roseola in phantom

The new medical transcriptionist, known for transcribing exactly what she hears, records "The location of the patient's abdominal pain is right up her quadrant."

Dictated – "patient to have sitz bath daily."
Transcribed – "patient to have six pack daily."

An 18-year-old student nurse was doing a case study on a 50-year-old gentleman who had undergone abdominal surgery. On the first postoperative day she was helping him walk around the room. He passed a little gas and said, "Oh I am so sorry."

As he was feeling rather embarrassed the nurse said, "Don't worry. That's just a feather in my cap," meaning he was getting good care and passing gas was a sign of recovery following the operation.

The patient said, "Well go stand by the door and I will make you an Indian Chief."

Two older men at a physiotherapy clinic were doing knee exercises. One turned to the other and inquired, "Old war injury?"

The second man replied, "Yeah. I'm old and it wore out."

Sign noted in a parking lot outside obstetrician/gynecologist office: "Deliveries only. 15 minute limit."

Announcement over the P.A. system at a gynecological clinic waiting room:

"To the owner of the red Vulva, your lights are on."

Sign in plastic surgeon's office:
"We make mountains out of mole hills."

Other medical disciplines have their own sense of humour...In order to communicate with patients it is necessary to get their attention. There is a story of the farmer who had a very stubborn donkey. In desperation the farmer consulted his vet. The vet arrived at the farm and said to the farmer, "You have to treat these animals with kindness. Get me a 2 x 4 six feet long." Armed with the club the vet rolled up his sleeves and approached the donkey. He raised the 2 x 4 and brought it down on the donkey's skull. The animal's knees buckled and his eyes rolled. The farmer was horrified. He protested to the vet, "I thought you said to treat them with kindness," to which the vet replied, "That's right, but first you have to attract their attention."

You never know who may be listening, even in the OR. Sometimes the patient hears more than you realize.

A woman was undergoing abdominal surgery, and due to a reaction to the anaesthetic had to be given extra oxygen. This had the unfortunate result of her regaining consciousness, albeit temporarily. The surgeon was singularly unimpressed and was heard to exclaim "Jesus Christ, what next?"

When the patient recovered and went home, her pastor came by to visit and to hear how the surgery had gone. She spoke of waking up part way through and said of the surgeon, "And he asked our Lord what to do next."

The pastor took but a moment to let out a most hearty laugh.

"Life is so short, the craft so long to learn."
*~ **Hippocrates** ~*

ISBN 1412078016